# TexasMonthly ON . . .
## FOOD

# TexasMonthly ON . . .

# FOOD

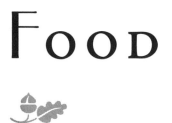

*From the editors of* TEXAS MONTHLY

INTRODUCTION BY EVAN SMITH
Editor, *Texas Monthly*

University of Texas Press ⬥ *Austin*

The recipes in "Stop and Smell the Lavender" are courtesy of Scott Cohen.

The recipe for drunken shrimp in "¡Viva Tequila!" is from *Tequila: The Book*, copyright © 1994 by Ann and Larry Walker (text) and Diane Borowski (illustrations). Used by permission of Chronicle Books, San Francisco.

The recipes for gazpacho macho and fiesta frijoles in "¡Viva Tequila!" are from *¡Tequila! Cooking with the Spirit of Mexico*, copyright © by Lucinda Hutson. Used by permission of the author.

The recipes in "Ladies, First" are reprinted from *Dining at the Governor's Mansion*, by Carl R. McQueary, by permission of the Texas A&M University Press, copyright © 2003 by Carl R. McQueary.

The recipes in "Got Game" are from *Fired Up: More Adventures & Recipes from Hudson's on the Bend*, by Jeff Blank and Sara Courington, copyright © 2005 by Laurentius Press.

Requests for permission to reproduce material from this work should be sent to:
    Permissions
    University of Texas Press
    P.O. Box 7819
    Austin, TX 78713-7819
    www.utexas.edu/utpress/about/bpermission.html

♾ The paper used in this book meets the minimum requirements of ANSI/NISO Z39.48-1992 (R1997) (Permanence of Paper).

Library of Congress Cataloging-in-Publication Data

Texas monthly on— food / from the editors of Texas monthly ; introduction by Evan Smith. — 1st ed.
    p.    cm.
    ISBN 978-0-292-71844-9 (pbk. : alk. paper)
    1. Diet—Texas.    2. Food habits—Texas.    3. Cookery—Texas.
I. Smith, Evan, 1966–    II. Texas monthly (Austin, Tex.)

TX360.U62T47    2008
641.59764—dc22

                                     2007034836

# CONTENTS

# INTRODUCTION

LIKE THE MAN SAID, we are what we eat. And, fortunately, what we eat is delicious. The cuisines of our state—Mexican food, barbecue, and comfort food by way of chicken-fried steak—have been the stuff of great meals for as long as there has been a Texas, and also of great magazine stories for as long as there has been a *Texas Monthly*. For 34 years now we've been telling our readers where to find and how to think about the best of everything, and nothing is more important to them, and to us, than the indigenous bests: the best burrito or margarita, the best brisket or beans, the best cream gravy or cornbread. Food has a constituency larger and more passionate than that of any other subject we cover; whoever you may be, wherever you live, it's also the thing that connects you to your neighbors down the block, across town, in the next county, and around the state. And food is fun to write about, though not always to report on: Ask our longtime restaurant critic and resident gourmand Patricia Sharpe to regale you with tales of eighty tacos in four days and you'll see why unlimited eating on someone else's dime may not be as enviable as it appears.

Pat has been, like a celebrated chef at a five-star restaurant, the one who's pulled the ingredients together masterfully, with grace and cheer, all these years. Many of the stories you're about to read originated with her, in conception or execution; others detoured through her office on their way to being served up to the more than

*Evan Smith*  two million readers who continue to hang on her every word. We and you owe her greatly for the impact she's had on all of our culinary lives. Thanks, Pat. You can keep the change.

🌸

*Evan Smith, Editor*
TEXAS MONTHLY
*August 2007*

# TexasMonthly on . . .
## Food

# FOOD CULTURE

# HOLY SHIITAKES!

 GARY CARTWRIGHT

Even though I love to cook, I never thought a grocery store could change my life. Central Market has—and twenty varieties of mushrooms are only one reason.

WHAT I LIKE TO DO when I'm not doing what I like to do best is eat. It follows that I also like to buy groceries and cook. Getting good groceries hasn't always been easy in Texas. Thirty years ago, if I had a recipe that required, say, pancetta, Parmigiano-Reggiano, and shiitake mushrooms, the easiest way to procure those ingredients was to fly to New York and take a cab to Balducci's. I was born to a generation for whom bread meant Mrs. Baird's white, and lettuce that didn't come from the garden was unfailingly iceberg. Chickens came from the chicken house out back, and extra-virgin olive oil was not something you talked about in mixed company. Then, in 1994, H-E-B, a grocery chain that I'd never thought of patronizing, changed my life by opening its first Central Market location on North Lamar Boulevard in Austin, a five-minute drive from my house.

Ever since, Central Market has been one of the poles on the axis of my life. Whole Foods is actually a few blocks closer, and I shop there too, but I've come to think of it as a smaller, less exciting, and more-organic-than-thou version of Central Market. The Central Market experience, you see, is without parallel. Every time I pull into the parking lot, which usually approaches gridlock, I feel that wonderful surge of childhood remembrances of sounds, smells, and possibilities unlimited: of Christmas morning or a circus pulling into town with lions, elephants, and clowns. There is a sense of apprehension too: the heart-pounding thrill of encountering the unknown. No wonder tour buses—tour buses!—stop out front. (A second Central Market is open in Austin, and there are locations in Houston, San Antonio, and the Metroplex, but the original stands alone. It's one of three places, along with the Capitol and the Bob Bullock state history museum, that Austinites take out-of-town guests.)

I bought a new car about the time Central Market opened. To date, it's got less than 30,000 miles on the odometer; my wife, Phyllis, jokes that I'm like the little old lady who drives only between her home and the church and grocery store. Okay, I also go to the gym and to the *Texas Monthly* office in downtown Austin, but you get an idea of the comfortable perimeter that Central Market has woven around my days. All that I need or desire is no more than a short drive away.

Shopping at Central Market is not for the timid. With its high ceilings and exposed girders, the building has the feel of a gigantic warehouse—a massive, pulsating sprawl of eatables, drinkables, accessories, and surprises. Adjusting to its chaotic flow takes practice and a Zen-like attitude on time and space. I have a friend who claims that he can't set foot inside without first ingesting a dangerous quantity of tranquilizers. Another friend boycotts the store because he refuses to master its checkout system, which expects shoppers to price produce and bulk purchases by punching four- or five-digit product codes into a scale. The system is an experiment in human honesty, because a shopper could easily fill a bag with expensive Kona coffee from Hawaii but use the code for much cheaper beans from Mexico; nobody would know the difference. Trust issues aside, some shoppers are simply confounded, creating traffic jams around the scales. I accept the travails of Central Market humbly, just as I accept the Texas heat or the inevitability of the Rangers finishing last in the Western Division.

Here's how I approach Central Market. First, I linger for a while outside, among the verdant explosion of flowering plants and clusters of chocolate mint, lemongrass, and Greek oregano. Breathing deeply, I close my eyes and allow the smells to calm my central nervous system. Guiding my grocery cart through the front door, I let myself be sucked into the belly of the beast, oblivious to the teeming masses jockeying for position with their bulging carts. I flit effortlessly around a produce section larger than most grocery stores and, it should be obvious by now, better-stocked. Red Dulce Mediterraneo peppers, Chinese cabbage, kiwano horned melons, taro roots, and jungles of leafy things compete for my attention. The selection of apples—fifty during the peak season of fall and early winter—nearly induces vertigo. In this rarefied environment, seasons vanish. Though it may be the dead of winter in Texas, the corresponding Chilean summer is perfect for peaches and plums, and Central Market has them air-lifted to Austin. A Central Market employee, or "partner," offers me slices of unbelievably sweet tree-ripened peaches. So numerous are the free samples that it is possible, theoretically, to eat three balanced meals a day without spending a penny.

I move serenely past long cases of iced-down fish, some with names I can't pronounce, passing many types and sizes of shrimp, whole baby octopuses, crab cakes, salmon cakes, and various marinades. Down the middle of the aisle that separates the seafood from an enormous meat counter are displays of bargain wines and tanks of live shellfish: lolling lobsters, restless Dungeness crabs, Cape Neddick and Rhode Island oysters, three varieties of clams, and wild Mediterranean black mussels. I've never learned to shuck oysters or pick crabs, but Central Market has guys who do that for me.

I walk in a dreamlike state past long rows of breads and cheeses, barrels of olives, bins of seasonings, salsas, sauces, dips, pizzas, quiches, beers, sausages, and mustards of the world. At a display of 1.5-liter bottles of Smart Water, with vapor-distilled electrolytes and a scale printed down one side of the package measuring how much smarter you get with each gulp, I pause to meditate on conspicuous consumption. By the time I reach the check-out station, I've chosen a jar of Texas 1015 Onion Glaze, a quart of freshly squeezed carrot-celery-beet-spinach juice, a bag of Chilean Kyoho grapes, four peaches, half a pound of Japanese squid salad, two filets of pepper-seared salmon with raspberry sauce, five small bags of assorted chile powders, a loaf of black Russian rye, two bottles of red Italian wine, and a small bouquet of pink tulips. The tab is $107.

A word about that wine: Though I buy by the case from my friend Greg Soechting at the Austin Wine Merchant, I can't resist browsing and inevitably grabbing one or two of the 2,800 selections stacked along the dark, cool corridors of Central Market's beer and wine section. Connoisseurs have learned to watch for the color-coded tags that designate wines favored by the members of the market's staff of tasters. "All of us are wine geeks," one explains. "We are passionate about wines. We study wines, read about them, talk about them." A taster might sample up to two hundred bottles a week. Recently I noticed a section reserved for "allocated wines," limited editions targeted to collectors, once relegated to the back room but lately made public. A collector I'm not, but this display is nevertheless fascinating. A bottle of Napa Valley 1999 La Sirena Cabernet, for example, is priced at $172. Eight years ago I bought a bottle of 1990 Niebaum-Coppola Rubicon for $35. Now it sells for $122.

To the caveat "Never go to the grocery store hungry," I would add: Never go to Central Market without a well-planned list. When you must choose from 500 varieties of cheese, 140 different olive oils, more than 40 kinds of coffee, and 20 varieties of mushrooms, discipline is essential. Unspoken is a threat: You break it, you buy it. Recently, I noticed a coffee called Jamaican Blue Mountain, priced at $39.99 a pound. A sign advised would-be purchasers to "please ask for assistance." No experiments in human honesty in that price range.

I can't help worrying that Central Market might eventually collapse under the weight of its own ambition. With such a vast and constantly changing inventory, spoilage must be a huge problem. Melissa Porter, the store's director of sales and marketing, acknowledges that it is. "We incur more of what we call 'shrink' than traditional stores," she told me. "To mitigate losses we use tools to predict demands and order the right amounts." I suspect that customers unknowingly share the burden of the shrink by paying dearly for such quality and freshness. But if you have to ask how much it costs, you shouldn't be shopping at Central Market.

One of the market's more devilish ploys is placing rows of fresh flowers by the checkout, so they're the last thing you see before leaving. This has proven useful in a way I never anticipated. Regarding that vague remark at the beginning of this column about what I like to do best, let me put it this way: Since the opening of Central Market, I've discovered that bringing home tulips helps it happen.

*June 2003*

# SOUR GRAPES

JORDAN MACKAY

Texas wines get no respect, and with good reason. But there is hope on the vine.

LAST YEAR AT A LIQUOR STORE in Austin a handwritten sign boldly trumpeted something that doesn't often get hyped in serious wine shops: "Texas Wine." Underneath it, in smaller print, undercutting the confidence of the pitch, was written: "We know what you're thinking, but trust us—this is a Texas wine actually worth trying." The wine being touted was from the first vintage of a recently founded Hill Country winery, Alamosa Wine Cellars, whose fourth and fifth vintages will be released October 1 to coincide with the beginning of Texas Wine month. But the real question was, Which was more odd, that a reputable wine store would admit to reservations about a wine or the existence of a Texas wine "actually worth trying"?

That Texas wines are often not good is the state's worst-kept secret. To be fair, Texas produces some good wines, but the vast majority of them are nothing that will turn heads. Of the forty wineries in Texas, only about five or six of them consistently put out decent wine. The thirty-odd others produce wines that, if they make an impression at all, it is usually a bad one. Even at a recent blind tasting at *Texas Monthly*, two $20 Cabernets—from Llano Estacado and Fall Creek, two fairly reliable producers—seemed thin and off-flavored compared with a $15 bottle from California.

Jordan
MacKay

The modern wine industry here, which proudly boasts that Texas is the fifth-largest wine-producing state in the country, has been in existence since the mid- to late seventies, roughly the same amount of time as the industries of Washington and Oregon (numbers three and four). Yet those two states regularly achieve wine that could be considered "world-class," meaning that it consistently receives high marks from the wine press and, because of scarcity caused by high demand and low production, generally fetches higher prices. Why is this important? Average wine does not sell an industry. "If you want to compete in the global or the national marketplace," says Thomas Matthews, the executive editor of *Wine Spectator*, "then you certainly need to make outstanding wines at a superpremium level with wide distribution and wide visibility."

Why has Texas yet to regularly produce great wine? It is axiomatic in the wine industry that good wine is made in the vineyard, which means that if you can grow excellent grapes, you can make excellent wine. Grape quality has thus far been the stumbling block in Texas. Texas viticulturists must grapple with an extreme climate that makes consistently good harvests difficult, intense heat that often makes the proper maturation of grapes impossible, and pressure from the market to grow popular grapes like Cabernet and Chardonnay even though they often do not do well here.

Greg Bruni, the winemaker at Lubbock's Llano Estacado, the winery generally credited with consistently producing the state's best wines, said that upon moving to Texas in 1993 from California, he was unprepared for the violence of Texas weather. "When I first got out here, I didn't know what a blue norther was," he says, reciting a litany of weather travails. "I had never experienced hail like that in the spring. Soils are spartan. We have extreme conditions. When it's hot, it's *really* hot. When it's cold, it's *really* cold. When it rains, it *really* rains."

Bruni, who made wine in California, is one of only a few Texas winemakers to have earned a degree at the University of California at Davis, considered to be the top winemaking school in the country, if not the world. But, he says, even that prestigious degree couldn't prepare him for the moody Texas climate. "California is a viticultural paradise," says the 47-year-old Bruni. "The grapes are so perfect that you would have to work to mess them up. But that's in a Mediterranean climate. Texas has a continental climate, which is a whole new ball game. They don't teach how to grow grapes in a Texas climate at school in California."

Excessive heat presents an especially difficult challenge. To develop the necessary components—flavors, aromas, tannins, acids, and colors—to make high-quality wine, grapes need to spend a certain amount of "hang time" maturing on the vine. It is during the maturation process, and its complex chemical reactions, that the flavor profiles of different grapes develop. For instance, immature Cabernet Sauvignon could make an herbaceous wine redolent of green pepper, while mature grapes will develop the more desirable cherry and cassis flavors and aromas associated with the best vinification of the grape. "In California," explains Bruni, "ripeness and maturity come often at the same time. But in Texas, because of the heat, ripeness comes before maturity." The dilemma Texas wine producers face is whether to harvest grapes that are ripe but still immature or to leave them on the vines past ripeness to develop maturity, thus risking spoilage and shrinkage. "We have to find a way for maturity to come sooner," says Bruni.

Some of the ripeness-maturity problem may occur because of the varieties of grapes being grown. Here, Texas winemakers find themselves in a unique bind. Wine in this country is marketed by grape type, as opposed to Europe, where wine is marketed by region of origin. American consumers typically shop for a varietal wine by name—a Cab or a Chard, they'll say, naming two of the most popular varieties—while in France, they will shop for a Burgundy or a Bordeaux to get roughly the same grapes. Texas wine producers find themselves in the pinch of having to produce and sell Cabernet, Chardonnay, and Merlot because that's what customers know. But they are probably not the grapes best suited to the Texas climate. There are other grapes, the so-called hot-weather varieties, that may grow better here.

One man who has invested himself in the hot-weather-variety theory is Jim Johnson, whose Alamosa Wine Cellars produced the bottles touted at the Austin liquor store. "If a grape is going to do well in Texas," says Johnson, "it's going to be something that's native to a warmer area, something like Syrah. It loves heat, and we've got plenty of heat." Johnson is giving Syrah, the great red grape of France's Rhône Valley, a try, as well as Tempranillo (the grape that produces famous wine from Spain's Rioja region), Sangiovese (the grape known principally for Chianti), and Viognier (the white grape of France's Rhône Valley). But the fact that these grapes have been able to produce world-class wines in the hotter climes of Europe doesn't necessarily mean they will in Texas: None of those European countries are as far south as Texas, which is in the same latitude as the North African countries of Algeria and Morocco. The risk, of course, is that no matter how good the wine is, consumers won't want it. How many times have you heard someone say, "I'm in the mood for a nice Viognier"?

But Johnson is unusual in that he has eschewed the conventional grapes and put his considerable investment into the ones with unfamiliar names. Like Bruni, Johnson is the rare Texas winemaker with a degree from UC-Davis. Unlike Bruni, Johnson is from Texas and didn't start his winemaking career until the age of 43. An affable fellow who wears a salt-and-red-pepper beard and brightly colored shirts, Johnson graduated from Davis and worked in California before heading back to Texas with a mission. "I left Texas to go to UC-Davis with the idea of eventually coming back, and part of that reasoning was that I had had some wines that made me think, 'Damn, I could do better than that.'"

Johnson bought 41 acres of land about 25 miles east of Lampasas, near the town of Bend. The decision to grow unconventional grapes was an easy one for him. "I think we can make great wine here," he says, "and I think when we do come up with something that's that good and world-class, it probably won't be Chardonnay and it isn't going to be Cabernet." So far his gamble seems to be paying off: This year's entire bottling of Tempranillo is already committed to retailers, and he expects the winery to turn a profit next year. That news will be encouraging to Greg Bruni, who has focused much of his energy on researching three or four hot-weather varietals. But he has to watch his bottom line and make the best wine he can from the Cabernet grapes the recalcitrant Texas soil gives him.

Hot-weather grapes may ultimately produce great wines here, but until then, Texas winemakers must deal with yet another obstacle: a shortage of viticultural talent. California has more than 800 wineries, and Oregon and Washington each have more than 150, compared with Texas's 40. More wineries mean a greater confluence of winemaking talent. And the talent simply doesn't flock to Texas like it does to the more temperate, wine-friendly climates of Washington and Oregon. "We first have to make some good wines to attract some people to Texas," says Johnson, "to show it can be done. Heck, if I hadn't been raised in Texas I probably wouldn't be here." That's part of the larger issue of critical mass: Lots of bad wine, it seems, is required to make one good wine. "California has more than eight hundred wineries," says Robert Parker, whose newsletter, *The Wine Advocate*, is arguably the most influential publication in the industry. "But once you get past the first six or seven dozen there, the quality is quite mediocre to actually insipid, probably no different than what you find across the board in Texas."

As it is, most of the strides made here toward producing world-class wine will be made by individuals like Johnson, who can afford (or who have risked everything trying to afford) bucking the market. Better wine is more expensive in part because it costs more to make it. A winemaker going for high quality will probably use French oak barrels, prized over American oak for its higher quality tannins but twice as expensive. Then, he or she must be able to leave the wine—a whole year's crop and the income that it represents—in those barrels for two years or more to age. These are significant expenses that cannot be shouldered by people or companies that can't afford to take a loss or wait to see a profit.

Richard Becker of Becker Vineyards is fortunate to have the resources to devote to making wine his way, relieving him of having to pander to the marketplace and the Texan palate. "We do not make a blush," says Becker, referring to the slightly sweet pink wines that are among the biggest sellers in the country and that are scoffed at by connoisseurs. "We make a completely dry Provincial-style rosé." At his Hill Country winery outside of Fredericksburg,

Becker makes wonderful wines of the same Cabernet, Chardonnay, and Merlot that have bedeviled other Texas growers as well as some unconventional wines like Viognier and Chenin Blanc, which are also excellent. He seems to have solved the maturation problem; each of his wines displayed remarkably good varietal characteristics (Cabernet that smelled of cassis, not green pepper) and had excellent color and a wonderful concentration of flavor, unlike many of the other Texan wines tasted. How does Becker do it? To let the Cabernet grapes reach maturation, he actually lets them become overripe on the vine. This means that they lose about 10 percent of their volume and their acidity drops. The volume is Becker's loss on his total production. He adds acid back in, a practice that is common in Texas. To get them at peak condition, he harvests at night, when it's cooler. And he invests in French oak and lets his wine spend a good deal of time there.

Johnson's wines, especially the Tempranillo and the Sangiovese, also show surprisingly good concentration and flavor. Llano's vast array yielded some excellent finds too, particularly its 1999 Passionelle, a Rhône-style blend, and its 1999 Riesling. Texas has also seen its first two $30 wines: Llano's Viviano and Fall Creek's Meritus. These are attempts to satisfy the growing demand for superpremium wine. Both are fine efforts but fall a little short; a better wine from Washington or California can be had for the money.

Clearly, though, the pursuit of a blockbuster wine is on. Even Leonard Garcia, the CEO of Ste. Genevieve, in Fort Stockton, assures that his winery—known primarily for jug wine—performs more than eighty trials a year, searching for that elusive combination of grape, soil, and growing practice that might produce a great wine. It will take that sort of commitment and investment to succeed.

"What you have in California, and you could say the same thing for France and Italy, are leaders," says Parker. "They are the locomotives for the industry. They get most of the publicity, make the best-quality wines, and tend to get most of the extravagant praise from the wine press. That creates a marketable image of Napa Valley or Sonoma, in California, or the Willamette Val-

ley, in Oregon. What you don't have is anybody like that in Texas.
That's the problem."

With winemakers like Bruni, Johnson, Becker, and others starting to figure things out, that may not be a problem much longer.

*October 2000*

# HOW THE WEST WAS WON OVER

SKIP HOLLANDSWORTH
AND PAMELA COLLOFF

Ⓢhe came. She saw. She put us on TV. And as the cattlemen's $12 million suit against Oprah Winfrey wore on, more and more Texans found themselves lining up on her side.

AS SHE STEPPED FROM HER GULFSTREAM JET, her two small cocker spaniels, Solomon and Sheba, nestled in her arms, Oprah Winfrey stopped for a moment and stared in silence at the treeless Panhandle horizon. She seemed stunned at what lay before her.

"Oprah!" shouted members of the news media from a roped-off area fifty yards away. From that distance, she looked like a great religious figure, her flowing brown pantsuit billowing in the wind like the robes of a prophet. The three local television stations cut into their regular programming to broadcast her arrival. "Oprah, how do you feel?" one of the reporters called out.

She hesitated for another moment, still staring at the unbroken flatness, and then turned to the cameras and offered her most cheerful wave. Escorted by bodyguards, she slipped into a black Chevrolet Suburban with black tinted windows, which raced her off to a meeting with her attorneys. "She's here!" an ecstatic Amarillo television reporter shouted into his microphone. "Oprah is here in Amarillo, and she has just waved right at us!"

Just when you thought that Texas was no longer Texas, just when you thought that we were finally becoming just like everyone

Skip
Hollandsworth
and
Pamela Colloff

else, something like the Oprah trial comes along. Who could have guessed that one of the most obscure and embarrassingly titled state laws on record—the False Disparagement of Perishable Food Products Act—would set off the most uproarious Texas range war since the fight over barbed wire? And, oh, what a glorious war, waged by a group of rich Texas cattle barons, the classic symbols of old frontier Texas, against an even richer black Chicago talk-show hostess, a classic symbol of modern-day American success. In ways that no one could have expected, the Oprah trial, involving a $12 million disparagement lawsuit over her April 1996 show about mad cow disease, became a battle for the heart and soul of the state. The cattle barons who filed the lawsuit saw themselves as Alamo-like defenders, hoping to save Texas from this contemporary Santa Anna who dared to say that she would never eat another hamburger. Winfrey, in turn, decided to counterattack with her best weapon: her own celebrity. She planned on turning Amarillo, the sagebrush kingdom, into Oprahrillo, broadcasting her daily show from the city during the trial's duration and even changing the show's name to *Oprah Winfrey in Texas*. "She's going to do her best to charm our pants off, and we all know she's good at it," grumbled Charles Rittenberry, a popular Amarillo trial lawyer, just before the trial began. "I don't know if our local cowboys are going to come out on top of this damn deal. We've already got wives of respectable ranchers sneaking around town, trying to get tickets to Oprah's show. I'm telling you, Oprah's about to cause a lot of hell to break loose out here."

Indeed, the Oprah trial was about to bring together an array of down-home West Texans and East Coast—educated lawyers, solemn *New York Times* reporters and bubbly *Entertainment Tonight* correspondents, bombastic vegetarian protesters, courthouse demonstrators wearing cow costumes, and even a marching kazoo band that stood outside the courthouse one bone-chilling winter day to play the *Andy Griffith Show* theme song, allegedly Winfrey's favorite tune. "We're all getting Oprah-itis; I can feel it in my bones," said Amarillo's famous millionaire eccentric, Stanley Marsh 3, the owner of a local television station and the creator of the display of half-buried cadillacs known as Cadillac Ranch. "By the time this thing is over, Texas is never going to be the same."

Excerpts from the *Oprah* mad cow episode have been rerun so many times that even people who don't watch daytime TV know them by heart. Howard Lyman, a failed Montana rancher turned vegetarian and animal rights activist, told Winfrey that American cattle were being fed ground-up meal made from dead livestock— the same practice that might have caused the spread of mad cow disease in Britain. ("Mad cow disease" is a brain-ravaging malady that has devastated cattle herds in Britain; in 1996 the British government announced that some humans may have died from eating beef contaminated by the disease.) Lyman argued that if the remains of one mad cow were fed to other cattle, thousands of cows, and in turn, countless American beefeaters, could be infected. As if on cue, Winfrey inquired, "You said this disease could make AIDS look like the common cold?" "Absolutely," Lyman replied, leading Winfrey to declare, "It has just stopped me cold from eating another burger!"

Cattle breeders are accustomed to beating back such elements as drought, dust storms, locusts, and twisters to get their cattle to market. But in the words of 71-year-old Bourdon R. Barfield, a descendant of a pioneer family in Amarillo, "Oprah was bigger than any whirlwind." On April 16, the very day her mad cow show aired, cattle futures prices on the Chicago Mercantile Exchange plunged. "Cattle prices had already been slipping somewhat," said Teel Bivins, an Amarillo state senator and veteran rancher, "but Oprah's show created a panic. The cattle market basically went into a free-fall." One Texas A&M economist said that in the three weeks following the Oprah show the cattle-feeding industry lost $87.6 million, although other observers blamed the loss on a devastating drought and an already volatile market shaken by Britain's mad cow scare.

Many of the nation's cattlemen—who with their vast ranches, cattle drives, and roundups had created some of the most enduring images of American mythology—felt whupped by a talkative "city woman." It wasn't, however, the fairest of fights. The show's producers cut out all but a few statements from a beef industry spokesman and a U.S. Agriculture Department expert on mad cow disease, both of whom insisted that American beef was safe. One of the show's producers later admitted that Winfrey had told an editor to "cut out the boring beef guy." Although she argued that she simply wanted to know why some cattle feeders were feeding cattle to cattle, her show did come off as rather alarmist. The reality was that the cattle industry had been moving away from such feed practices. And there had never been a documented case of mad cow disease in the U.S.

The cattlemen wanted revenge. But which of them dared to take on Oprah, the highest-paid entertainer in the world, once described on the cover of *Life* as "America's most powerful woman"?

Enter Paul Engler, a native Nebraskan who had moved to the Panhandle in 1960 with one simple, albeit unglamorous, vision: to make cows fatter, faster. He envisioned fenced-in commercial feedlots stretching across the Panhandle where cattle would while away their last days by the feed trough. The notion eventually made him a multimillionaire and one of the most powerful cattlemen in the country. The 68-year-old Engler is all-male, as tough as a fence post; a framed photo of a double-barreled shotgun, permanently cocked at visitors, hangs over his desk. He's known as a bit of a hellion; he once got so furious upon hearing himself called a farmer on television that he told his attorney, "If that guy calls me a farmer again, you sue his ass."

"Engler could be one of John Wayne's pals," said Stanley Marsh. "He shakes your hand real hard, and for kicks, he'll take you way up in the air in his helicopter and show you this real pretty lake on his property that looks yellow in the sunlight. When the helicopter gets lower, you realize it's a lake of cow piss coming from his feedlots."

Engler and three smaller Amarillo cattle feeders filed suit in federal court under the False Disparagement of Perishable Food Products Act, a 1995 law that states that those who interfere with the sale of Texas produce by knowingly making false statements can be held liable to the producer for damages. The lawsuit seemed flimsy at best. Winfrey's announcement that she was swearing off beef was clearly protected by the First Amendment. And even if the show was flagrantly biased against cattlemen, at least some airtime had been given to the beef proponents. Furthermore, it was going to be difficult to pin the cattlemen's finan-

cial losses (Engler said he had lost $6.7 million) directly on Win-
frey, since beef prices had already been declining. And then there
was the question of whether a law designed to protect perishable
produce could be applied to livestock. "It's questionable just how
perishable a thousand-pound steer really is," quipped Winfrey's
attorney, Chip Babcock of Dallas.

Standing in one of his wind-whipped feedlots last December, Engler said indignantly from beneath the brim of his white
Stetson, "The picture presented on that show was that people in
the beef industry were picking up dead cows in the middle of the
night, tossing them in the back of their pickups, slicing them up,
and then dumping bloody cow parts into feed troughs." His cattle
stood quietly in the mud, blinking slowly under their long lashes
and chewing their feed. "Exaggerations, untruths, and innuendo,"
he bellowed, flashing his thick gold ring emblazoned with a C of
diamonds in honor of his company, Cactus Feeders. At the time,
his desk was littered with fan letters and checks from ranchers
from all over the country. Politicians also got into the act: The
state's agriculture commissioner, Rick Perry, told Engler to "go
over and blow the hell out of them." Engler knew that if he won
his lawsuit, he would be considered one of the greatest cattlemen
in Texas history, next to Charles Goodnight. "Let's face it, some of
the best days of Amarillo's cowboy life are long gone," said Charles
Rittenberry, "so here was our chance for one last hurrah."

Many lawyers figured the case would never get to trial, but
late last year federal judge Mary Lou Robinson ruled the suit
was valid, and then she shocked Winfrey's attorneys by announc-
ing that an impartial jury could be seated in Amarillo. The irony
seemed too delicious to be true. Oprah was going to be forced to
spend at least a month in Amarillo, the board game—flat beef
capital of Texas—a city that has been known to smell like a cow
patty when the wind comes out of the east and wafts through the
stockyards on its way downtown. Yeehaw! Amarillo! The shoot-
out was on.

By the time most of the news media began showing up in Amarillo in late January for the trial, the city of 175,000 was close to
pandemonium. "My God, everybody's trying to figure out how to

get on the jury," said a local attorney. "I've even heard there are some women wanting to get on the jury just so they can pose nude for *Playboy* the way that O. J. Simpson juror did."

During the first week of the trial, a dozen satellite television trucks circled the federal courthouse like a bunch of covered wagons, while national reporters fanned out through the city, looking for cowboys and rednecks and steak eaters. The coverage, of course, was not flattering. An Amarillo columnist said the national media had made Amarillo look like "a tumbleweed-strewn nest of yokels." Kent Harrell, the news director of Amarillo television station KVII, was asked by the producer of a call-in radio talk show in New York whether there was a reporter at the station with a thick Texas drawl who could talk in a rustic way about the upcoming trial. Harrell said he had no such reporters: "We speak regular English out here."

It was hard to believe that something or someone could interfere with Amarillo's allegiance to beef. This, after all, is a city the cattlemen built. The lobby of the federal courthouse, where Winfrey would be put on trial, is ringed with a sweeping mural of a cattle drive. Amarillo's largest private employer, with 3,300 workers, is the Iowa Beef Processors' slaughterhouse. One of the city's most famous landmarks is the Big Texan Steak Ranch, which offers a 72-ounce steak (four and a half pounds) free if a customer can eat it and all the trimmings in an hour. Within 150 miles of Amarillo, six million head of cattle, a third of the nation's cattle supply, are fattened in feedlots. All of which would explain those fire-red bumper stickers proclaiming "The Only Mad Cow in Amarillo is OPRAH" that dotted the city. To show his support for Panhandle cattlemen, Gary Molberg, Amarillo's chamber of commerce president, issued an internal memo in early January admonishing the chamber's staff not to attend Winfrey's show while it was broadcasting in Amarillo nor to give her or her production company "any red carpet rollouts, key to the city, flowers."

But then came a major defection from the ranks of Amarillo's power structure. Nancy Seliger, the spunky wife of Amarillo mayor Kel Seliger, sent Winfrey a handwritten note inviting her to a meeting of Seliger's book club. Every woman in Amarillo knew within days what happened next: Winfrey immediately picked up the phone, called Mrs. Seliger, graciously thanked her, and chatted with her for several minutes about—among other things—where to get her hair done in Amarillo.

Although Engler was no longer talking to the press—the judge had slapped a gag order on all potential witnesses and lawyers involved in the case—the word was that he and his cohorts were dismayed that one of Amarillo's finer women would cross the line. ("We are proud of the town our cattlemen built," said Nancy Seliger, "but there was no sense in being rude.") One can only guess how Engler reacted when phone lines across the Panhandle temporarily shut down one afternoon after an 800-number advertising tickets to tapings of *Oprah* in Amarillo flashed across television screens. A spokesman for the show said 215,000 calls came in within thirty minutes.

What had happened? Instead of creating a groundswell of support for cattlemen, the industry's practices were being scrutinized more closely than ever by the media. Ralph Nader wrote a column, printed in newspapers around the country, comparing the cattlemen's suit with King George III's attempts to silence Americans. Other writers said that Engler's lawsuit threatened the First Amendment. The *Dallas Morning News* received letters calling Engler and his supporters "crybaby cattlemen" and "spoiled children."

"People in the beef industry," said one insider, "are saying off the record that this is a public relations disaster." In an early survey the *Amarillo Globe-News* found that 1,284 of its responding readers thought Winfrey would win, while only 280 thought the cattleman would. Agriculture commissioner Perry, a gung ho backer of the lawsuit, was conspicuously quiet about it—maybe because he was running for lieutenant governor. By mid-January, the fire-red bumper stickers seemed to have thinned out, outnumbered by "Amarillo Loves Oprah" T-shirts. When Gary Molberg, the hapless chamber of commerce president, realized just what support there was for Winfrey in Amarillo—some residents were lining up alongside a remote highway before dawn in the bitter cold simply to watch her jog—he issued a retraction of his memo and sent her a bouquet of yellow roses.

Not that she needed him. The first week of the trial made it clear that there were a lot of Amarillans who worshiped Oprah. Every morning, just for her benefit, one local television station reported the temperature in Chicago, while another offered a daily sight-seeing tip just for her. One television reporter gave a sincere look at the camera and said, "Oprah, if you're watching, please come down to the station, and we'll talk about anything you wish!" Almost every morning when she arrived at the courthouse in her black Suburban, a throng of female fans raced down the sidewalk to get a better look at her. "We love you, Oprah!" they screamed. "We love you!" Winfrey was forbidden to speak about the suit, but she knew how to get attention. When she left at the end of the day, she always rolled down the window of the car, stuck her head out, and smiled benevolently at everyone. When her getaway was halted at one point by an inopportune red light, fans stormed the street, mobbing the car. "Jesus, you'd think it was the president and his intern in there," one Amarillo cop muttered to another by the barricades.

Other than reporters, few spectators even recognized Engler as he strode in and out of the courthouse. One afternoon the great cattleman, known in the industry as the Father of the Feedlots, found himself walking past 150 people who had gathered to serenade Winfrey with kazoos. A chagrined Engler slouched under his Stetson, crossed Taylor Street, and disappeared around the next corner as the kazoos buzzed merrily behind him. The sole vocal demonstrator for Engler's group was a rather obnoxious man who, over the din, frantically shouted, "Eat more beef!" "I have no doubt that Engler thought he was walking into a hometown court and putting a foreigner on trial," said Jeff Blackburn, an Amarillo attorney who had been used by CNN as an expert commentator on the Oprah trial. "To these cattlemen, Oprah—a successful black woman from Chicago—seems like a foreigner. But the real comeuppance is that Engler is a lot more foreign to people here than Oprah. People in Amarillo watch *Oprah* every day."

And to keep everyone watching, Winfrey made sure that her shows, taped at the Amarillo Little Theatre, were filled with extravagant salutes to the very place she was being accused of ruining. "Get ready for Oprah, Texas-style!" the announcer would say at the beginning of each show, and from behind the curtain would come Oprah, grinning like a rodeo queen. Her first show included two native Texans, country music singer Clint Black and movie star Patrick Swayze, who gave her a cowboy hat and a pair of black Lucchese boots and then two-stepped with her around the stage. There were pre-taped clips of Texas celebrities, such as LeAnn Rimes and Kenny Rogers, welcoming Oprah to Texas. Other shows celebrated all things big in Texas, including gigantic mansions, huge ranches, big hair, big purses, and multimillionaire bachelors who were looking for that perfect gal. Winfrey loved talking with a fake countrified Texas accent, using phrases such as "How are y'all?" and "Did you now?" and "That's where the rubber hits the road, I reckon." At some point in every show she would mention how nice she found the people of Amarillo. Under the colored lights, at the lip of the stage, they beamed back at her.

Despite the bedlam outside the courtroom, there was still a decent possibility that Engler and his fellow cattlemen could win inside. The all-white jury included a woman who had been involved in cattle feeding 25 years ago and a descendant of one of Amarillo's oldest ranching families. The jurors sat through laborious testimony—involving carcass weights, commodities markets, and the difference between feeder cattle and fed cattle—as many spectators nodded off. When Engler's son mixed up a bunch of cattle feed in a barrel before the jury, Winfrey looked nauseated. Otherwise, she did an admirable job of looking interested, scribbling notes on her legal pad and listening intently to discussions about slaughterhouse quotas and the "scrapie control program."

Engler's attorneys put up a good fight, proving that he had long ago stopped using ground-up meat meal at his feedlots and showing how slipshod the editing of the mad cow episode had been. There was testimony from the beef expert whom Winfrey had told after the first show, "We weren't fair to you," and from a government expert on mad cow disease who said there was "a snowball's chance in hell" that mad cow disease would ever strike the U.S. Later he broke down in tears as he recalled his attempts to defend beef on the show, describing the perky female audience as a "lynch mob."

Then, midway through the third week of the trial, as a cold, thick fog rolled in over the city, it was Winfrey's turn to talk. She ascended the courthouse stairs among a cluster of U.S. marshals, clutching the hand of her close friend, poet Maya Angelou. Outside the courthouse, her fans—including a man in a cow suit and a woman holding a sign that read "U Are Loved"—held a silent vigil in the below-freezing temperatures. Inside, after Angelou whispered some encouraging words in her ear, Winfrey rose slowly from her seat and walked to the witness stand. Spectators in the packed courtroom sucked in their breath. The moment of truth had arrived.

Engler's persistent attorney, Joseph Coyne, began by taking her through the entire transcript of the show, line by excruciating line, slowly picking apart each word. He pointedly asked about her decision to swear off beef and grilled her about her show's anti-beef agenda. Winfrey's patience with Coyne quickly wore thin: She sighed loudly, restlessly tossed her black hair over her shoulder, and cast sidelong glances at her legal team. But Coyne bore in, accusing her of negligence for not double-checking Howard Lyman's claims or remedying her producer's careless editing. After one particularly insistent line of repetitive questioning, Winfrey paused, peered at the lawyer, leaned in to the microphone, and in a thrilling, low voice, thundered: "Mr. Coyne, I provide a forum for people to express their opinions. . . . *This is the United States of America.* We are allowed to do this in the United States of America." It was as if an electric current suddenly ran through the courtroom. Spectators who had slouched for hours on the court's hardwood benches suddenly straightened up, craning to get a better view of the witness box. Reporters scribbled in their notepads while the cattlemen's wives nudged each other anxiously.

By the time Winfrey's attorney took the floor, the talk-show queen's tone had taken on the air of a revival-meeting sermon. "I am a black woman in America, having gotten here believing in a power greater than myself," she intoned in response to a question about her integrity. "I cannot be bought. I answer to the spirit of God that lives in us all." She recounted her penniless beginnings in backwater Mississippi and her hardscrabble rise to fame, which began with her winning first place in Nashville's Miss Fire Prevention contest when she was seventeen. As spectators hung on her

every word, she chronicled her triumphs over childhood abuse,
racism, obesity, and poverty to become one of the wealthiest, most
influential women in the world. Paul Engler shifted uneasily in
his chair. Was it possible that he and his fellow plaintiffs were
thinking—as others in the courtroom certainly were—that this
black urban woman embodied all the rugged, heroic qualities that
we used to look for in the great Texas men of the past, men who
had tamed the vast frontier? Men who believed they could accomplish anything? Men who didn't need lawyers to help them earn
a living? Winfrey turned and looked directly at the twelve jurors
who were soon to judge her. "I am in this courtroom to defend my
name," she said. "I feel in my heart I've never done a malicious act
against any human being."

There were still plenty of other witnesses to be heard—the
trial was expected to last through the end of February—but many
Amarillo lawyers who had been following the case figured Engler
was sunk. No one around town appeared particularly upset. The
cattlemen were still making money. People were still eating beef.
And the citizens had other things to think about, namely getting
home early from work so they could catch Oprah's show. Every
night the Amarillo Little Theatre was invaded by Amarillans who
wanted to see Oprah and hear her talk with her fake Texas accent.
They loved the Texas that she had recreated for them—a Texas
with a golden, nostalgic glow, a Texas where everyone was friendly
and funny, larger than life, and able to ride a horse. The fact that
her mythological Texas had little connection to reality didn't seem
to matter. Indeed, at the end of every one of her shows, Texans
stood and roared their approval, prouder than ever of who they
thought they were.

*March 1998*

# STOP AND SMELL
# THE LAVENDER

### PATRICIA SHARPE

Groves of olive trees. Acres of vineyards. Herds of goats yielding tangy cheese. Is this Texas or the South of France? Nowadays, the foods and flavors of Provence can be found a lot closer to home. Here's where—plus recipes *TRÈS DÉLICIEUSES*.

IT HAPPENED THE FIRST TIME I visited the South of France. My boyfriend and I were nuzzling our way through the countryside in a rented Renault when suddenly the same idea struck us like a bolt of summer lightning. Seldom had we felt so close, so in tune. Gazing deeply into each other's eyes, we asked the wordless question: "What are all these rolling hills, limestone bluffs, oak trees, and prickly-pear cacti doing in *France?*" No, we hadn't been mysteriously teleported back to Texas: Provence is a dead ringer for the Hill Country.

Until recently, though, the resemblance stopped with the terrain. The singular *terroir* of Provence—the character of the land that manifests itself in the region's wine, olives and olive oil, herbs, lavender, goat cheese, lamb, and honey—had no homegrown counterpart. But all that has changed in the past decade, as a gaggle of entrepreneurs—some starry-eyed, some sharp-eyed—has started transforming the local landscape. So one balmy week this spring, I hit the road to find out what's happening in the mythical region of Provence, Texas.

Just outside the town of Dripping Springs (affectionately called

"Drippin'" by the natives), I turned off the main highway and followed narrow country roads to the sixty-acre farm where Sara and Denny Bolton have been making their prize-winning Pure Luck goat cheese for ten years. After being nibbled and drooled on by a herd of pushy female goats, I went with Sara's daughter and fellow cheesemaker Amelia Sweethardt into the spotless small building where the cheese is produced. As I asked questions and generally got in her way, she scooped and packaged creamy white mounds of chèvre. Pure Luck's main product is fresh goat cheese, both plain and flavored (I love the chipotle), but it also turns out five other types, including a piquant, log-shaped Sainte Maure and Del Cielo, a lusciously soft aged version that's similar to Camembert. On most weekends and holidays, you can wander around the farm, pet the goats, and buy cheese on the honor system from a tiny hut across the road. You might even come home with an armful of fresh flowers too, since Pure Luck also grows snapdragons, zinnias, larkspur, and a dozen other species.

Out at Hill Country Lavender, owners Jeannie Ralston and Robb Kendrick had been praying to the rain gods to stop, to no avail: Their fields of lavender were green, not purple. "It's the cool, wet weather," Ralston said, looking a little frazzled. "The plants are way behind schedule." Ever since she and Kendrick—who are married—visited a lavender farm on a trip to France, they've been obsessed with raising it themselves. "We put in two thousand plants in 1999," she said. Now they have six thousand on their 225-acre place near Blanco. As the three of us surveyed the rows of clumpy gray-green shrubs fanning out in every direction, Ralston predicted that by late June the plants would be heavy with flowers and the air thick with lavender's pungent aroma. On weekends from mid-May to early July (if the weather cooperates), hordes of lavender lovers show up and pay $4 a bunch to cut their own. The rest of the year, visitors can wander around the fields and investigate the farm's rustic gift shop, which is stuffed with oils, candles, sachets, and other fragrant items. "People are crazy for lavender," said Ralston.

It used to be that the words "Texas wine" elicited snorts of disbelief. Now "Texas olive oil" is having the same effect. But contrary to expectations, olive trees are thriving in Texas. Some half dozen incurable optimists are convinced that Texas olive oil is the next big thing, and the one who has gone the farthest the fastest is Dallas businessman Jim Henry, the owner of the Texas Olive Company. In ten years the gentleman farmer and his wife, Kathy, have planted 40,000 olive trees in the sandy soil of South Texas. When I first saw the skinny little saplings standing bravely on the flat-as-a-tortilla plains outside Carrizo Springs, I was taken aback: Instead of the gnarled, Van Gogh trees I had envisioned, here were tidy, drip-irrigated rows of upright trunks. But if they last long enough, these trees will be geezers too someday. This year will mark the Henrys' first big production—they hope to turn out around five thousand bottles of olive oil.

If olive oil is one of the newest Provence-style products in Texas, honey is one of the oldest. Fain's Honey, of Llano, for instance, has been around for 78 years. Second-generation-owner Dewey Fain and his wife, Erwinna, met me at their honey-production plant on Texas Highway 16, where he proceeded to give me a crash course in honeymaking. It was more fun than a grade-school field trip. We started at the magnolia tree in front of the building, where we watched a few random bees packing pollen into the little saddlebags on their legs. Then we hopped into Fain's truck and drove five miles down the road to check on some of his hives (he has others in South Texas). The sky was overcast, so the bees were cranky—they like sunny weather—and Fain insisted I wear a white bee suit that made me look a lot like the Michelin tire man. "Africanized bees have taken a lot of the fun out of beekeeping," he said. "These days I won't go near a hive without a bee suit on." The tour ended back in his seven-hundred-square-foot honey-processing room, where as many as two hundred 55-gallon barrels of natural raw honey are bottled every year. Fain's honey distills a summer's worth of wildflowers, mesquite, catclaw, cactus, wild persimmon, guajillo, and beebrush into a subtly spicy blend he calls Texas brush honey.

The Francofication of Texas doesn't stop with lavender, goat cheese, olive oil, and honey. Lamb is the red meat of the South of France, and Ranchers' Lamb, in San Angelo, has been selling chops, racks, loins, shanks, and more—all grain-fed—for six years. Near Fredericksburg, Becker Vineyards is making a dry rosé called Provençal, which is like the wine that is the summer drink of choice in southern France. (Becker also sells dried lavender, for a Provençal twofer.) And finally, herb growers all around Texas, such as the Fredericksburg Herb Farm, are raising the fresh rosemary, thyme, tarragon, basil, sage, lavender, and more that are the region's indispensable seasoning mix: *herbes de Provence*.

Of course, it's one thing to know about all the foods that make up this bounty. It's quite another to know what to do with them, which is why we turned to San Antonio chef Scott Cohen for help. A transplanted New Yorker, Cohen not only trained in French techniques but also completed a demanding apprenticeship program known as a *stage* in—you guessed it—Provence. Eighteen years ago, though, he married a Texan and is now a complete nut about seeking out Texas-raised foods to use in his highly regarded restaurant, Las Canarias, at La Mansión del Rio Hotel. Who better, we thought, to put together a Provençal feast, Texas style?

## DIRECTORY

### GOAT CHEESE

Fresh and dry, aged goat cheese available at the *Mozzarella Company*, 2944 Elm, Dallas; 800-798-2954, mozzco.com. Closed Sunday. Also available at many supermarkets. Fresh goat cheese available at *Pure Luck*, 101 Twin Oaks Trail, Dripping Springs; 512-858-7034, purelucktexas.com. From the intersection of U.S. 290 and Ranch Road 12, go 3.6 miles west on 290; turn right on McGregor Lane, proceed for 1.7 miles, turn left on Martin Road, and continue .6 mile to the farm stand, just before Twin Oaks Trail. The farm is a few hundred feet farther on Martin Road (turn right at the first gravel driveway past the farm stand). Open weekends and some holidays if the sign is out on 290 at McGregor Lane. Pure Luck cheese also available at some Central Market and Whole Foods stores.

### HERBS

*Fredericksburg Herb Farm*, 407 Whitney, Fredericksburg; 800-259-4372, fredericksburgherbfarm.com. From Main Street, turn south on Milam and go 6 blocks to Whitney. Open daily.

## HONEY

*Fain's Honey,* 3744 S. Texas Highway 16, Llano; 325-247-4867, fainshoney.com. From the intersection of Texas highways 71 and 16, go 1.5 miles south on 16; the store is on the left. Closed weekends, except by appointment. Honey also available at some H-E-B, Central Market, Whole Foods, Sun Harvest, Super S, and other stores.

## LAVENDER

*Hill Country Lavender,* 1672 McKinney Loop, Blanco; 830-833-2294, hillcountrylavender.com. From the traffic light on U.S. 281 in downtown Blanco, go west on FM 1623 for 2.5 miles; turn right on County Road 106 (McKinney Loop), and continue for 1.5 miles. Open weekends through Christmas. Closed January through March. Dried lavender is also available at Becker Vineyards (see below).

## OLIVE OIL

*Texas Olive Company,* Carrizo Springs. Not open to the public. Available by mail order in October: 214-325-5787 or olivehenry@aol.com.

## ROSÉ WINE

*Becker Vineyards,* 464 Becker Farms Road, 830-644-2681, beckervineyards.com. From Fredericksburg, go about 11 miles east on U.S. 290, then turn right on Jenschke Lane. Open daily. Becker Provençal rosé available only at the vineyard; other Becker wines available in many supermarkets and liquor and wine stores.

## RECIPES

### MESCLUN, FENNEL, AND CANDIED-PECAN SALAD WITH LEMON-BASIL DRESSING

#### Lemon-Basil Dressing

1 bunch fresh basil
1 shallot, coarsely chopped
6 tablespoons champagne vinegar
2 tablespoons fresh lemon juice
2 eggs

¾ cup salad oil
¼ cup Texas extra-virgin olive oil
salt and white pepper to taste

In a food processor, purée first 5 ingredients. Slowly add oils and process until incorporated. Season with salt and pepper. Dressing should be thin enough to lightly coat salad greens; if too thick, thin with cool water.

### Salad

1 tablespoon sugar
1 cup chopped pecans
pinch cayenne pepper
1 bulb fennel
4 ounces firm, aged Texas goat cheese or
    Parmigiano-Reggiano
4 cups mesclun (such as arugula, dandelion greens, frisée,
    mizuma, oak leaf lettuce, radicchio, and sorrel), as small
    and young as possible
16 red cherry or pear tomatoes, halved
Lemon-Basil Dressing (recipe above)
salt and freshly ground pepper to taste

Preheat oven to 200 degrees. Toss sugar, pecans, and cayenne with 1 teaspoon water. Place nuts on an ungreased cookie sheet and toast for 20 minutes; set aside. Shave fennel paper-thin (use a mandoline for best results) and keep in ice water until ready to use. Shave cheese paper-thin. Toss candied pecans, mesclun, and tomatoes with ½ to ¾ cup dressing. Adjust seasoning. Divide greens evenly among 8 plates and top with fennel and cheese. Serves 8.

### HONEY-MUSTARD LAMB WITH RED WINE LAVENDER JUS

### Lamb

2 boneless Texas lamb loins, about 1 pound each, trimmed
salt to taste
1 teaspoon freshly ground pepper

1 teaspoon dried *herbes de Provence*
1 teaspoon Texas honey
1 teaspoon Dijon mustard
1 teaspoon whole-grain mustard
2 tablespoons Texas extra-virgin olive oil

Cut lamb into 8 equal portions, and rub with salt, pepper, and *herbes de Provence*. Combine honey and mustards. To cook lamb medium-rare, heat olive oil over high heat in a 12-inch sauté pan until oil is lightly smoking. Reduce heat to medium high and cook lamb for 3 minutes on first side. Turn, brush cooked side with honey mustard, and cook for 3 minutes. Turn again, brush with honey mustard, and cook for 15 seconds. Remove meat from pan, wrap in foil, and keep warm until ready to serve. Remove juices (if any) from pan and reserve pan and juices for sauce (skim off excess grease).

### Sauce

1 cup red wine, such as Cabernet Sauvignon
½ teaspoons fresh Texas lavender buds (a little less if using dried lavender buds, available in bulk spice section)
salt and freshly ground pepper to taste
about 1 cup demi-glace (homemade, or make from packaged demi-glace concentrate, often stocked with soup mixes)
½ cup microgreens (baby lettuces and herbs) for garnish (optional)

Place lamb pan over high heat and deglaze with wine. Add lavender buds and lightly season with salt and pepper. Reduce wine to ¼ cup. Add enough prepared demi-glace to the reserved lamb juices (if any) to make 1 cup and return to pan. Reduce to ½ cup. Let cool until grease rises to top; skim off grease with a spoon or ladle and strain sauce. Keep warm until ready to serve.

### To serve:

Cut each portion of lamb into 3 slices, arrange attractively on 8 plates, and drizzle with sauce. Serve with South Texas Ratatouille and garnish plate with microgreens. Serves 8.

Patricia
Sharpe

SOUTH TEXAS RATATOUILLE

1 white onion, diced

½ cup Texas extra-virgin olive oil

6 medium cloves garlic, minced

1 large eggplant, peeled and cut into *batons* (sticks) ¼ inch by
 ¼ inch by 2 inches

1 small zucchini, cut into *batons* (as above)

1 small yellow squash, cut into *batons* (as above)

1 small chayote, peeled and cut into *batons* (as above)

½ small jicama, peeled and cut into *batons* (as above)

1 small red bell pepper, seeded and cut into *batons* (as above)

1 small yellow bell pepper, seeded and cut into *batons* (as
 above)

1 small poblano chile, seeded and cut into *batons* (as above;
 you do not need to roast or remove skin)

4 beefsteak or other ripe tomatoes, diced

½ to ¾ cup chopped flat-leaf parsley, basil, cilantro, and
 Mexican oregano

sprigs of fresh herbs such as basil, flat-leaf parsley, cilantro,
 and Mexican oregano (including oregano flowers) for
 garnishing plate; tear off 4 or more whole basil leaves per
 person to scatter on top of each serving of ratatouille

salt and freshly ground pepper to taste

In a large pot, sauté onion in olive oil over high heat for about 1 minute, being careful not to burn. Add garlic and cook until very light brown. Stirring to keep from burning, add eggplant, zucchini, and yellow squash and cook for 3 minutes. Add chayote and jicama and cook for 2 minutes. Add peppers and poblano and cook for 2 minutes. Finally, add tomatoes and herb mixture and cook for 2 minutes. Season with salt and pepper. Most of the vegetables should be between al dente and soft, though the eggplant may be a bit mushy.

### To serve:

Put on plates with lamb and top with basil leaves. Garnish plates with sprigs of other herbs. Serves 8.

*HONEY-LAVENDER ICE CREAM*

2 cups milk
2 cups cream
6 tablespoons sugar, divided into 2 equal batches
¼ cup Texas honey
1 teaspoon dried lavender buds, available in bulk spice
    section
8 large egg yolks

In a saucepan over medium heat, scald milk, cream, half of sugar, and honey (do not boil; if using a candy thermometer, bring to a temperature of 180 degrees). Remove from heat, add lavender, cover, and let infuse for about 15 minutes. In a large bowl, briefly whisk together yolks and remaining sugar. Gradually whisk milk mixture into yolks.

Put in a saucepan and cook over medium-high to high heat, stirring rapidly with a heat-resistant rubber spatula, until mixture coats spatula or reaches 180 degrees on a candy thermometer; do this step as quickly as possible. Immediately strain mixture into a stainless-steel bowl and cool bowl in ice water for at least 20 minutes. Pour into an ice cream machine and follow manufacturer's instructions. Makes 1 ½ quarts.


*GOAT CHEESE SAMPLER WITH TEXAS TAPENADE*

2 cups pitted niçoise olives or other French black olives
¼ cup Texas extra-virgin olive oil
1 anchovy filet
1 teaspoon capers
1 teaspoon pickled nopalitos, available at many supermarkets,
    including H-E-B and Central Market (or omit and double
    amount of capers)
1 sprig fresh thyme, leaves only, chopped
1 teaspoon sherry vinegar
salt and freshly ground pepper to taste
selection of Texas goat cheeses, about 1 pound in all
1 baguette, sliced

a few sprigs fresh *herbes de Provence* (such as lavender,
    marjoram, rosemary, sage, summer savory, basil, and
    thyme) for garnish (optional)
Texas rosé wine

### Make Texas Tapenade:

In a food processor, pulse olives just until coarsely chopped.
Add olive oil, anchovy, capers, nopalitos, thyme, vinegar, salt,
and pepper, and pulse until mixture forms a loose paste. Do not
overprocess.

### To serve:

Put a bowl of Texas Tapenade on a platter and surround with goat
cheeses. Arrange slices of baguette around edge and garnish platter with sprigs of herbs. Accompany with Texas rosé. Serves 8.

*July 2004*

# WAR FARE

PATRICIA SHARPE

Surviving for 48 hours on a diet of "meals ready to eat" gave me a taste of military life—and a new respect for Tabasco sauce.

THE EDITOR OF THIS MAGAZINE is trying to kill me.

Oh, I know what you're thinking: "Come on, that can't be right. Why, Evan Smith seems so nice, a family man and all. Whatever could make you think he has it in for you?"

But I swear it's true. How else am I to interpret his twisted response to the story idea I suggested a few weeks ago, not long after I saw a mention in the newspaper that a Texas business—the Wornick Company, of McAllen—is one of three companies in the country that assemble and package portable meals for soldiers in places like Afghanistan?

"I've read that story before," Evan said.

"You've read about the *humanitarian* food," I told him, a bit testily. "The military meals are different. And they aren't made just for the armed services. Ordinary people can get them at military-surplus stores and over the Internet. Our readers could get them to take on camping trips; they could stock them in their basement survival bunkers; they could . . ."

Suddenly a wicked little smile began to play about Evan's lips. "Okay, Pat," he said. "You can do this story, but I want you to eat nothing but MREs for forty-eight hours. Review them like you would a restaurant and write them up." And that is how I found myself sitting on the floor of a local military-surplus store in front of a bin of "meals ready to eat" (MREs, as they're generally called), trying to decide whether I wanted to shuffle off this mortal coil with menu number 2 (boneless pork chop) or menu number 17 (beef teriyaki).

*Meal 1, dinner.* I have snipped open the 8- by 12.5-inch, tan, heavy-duty plastic pouch containing menu number 9 and arranged the contents on my kitchen counter: a packet of beef stew (moist, not freeze-dried); two large crackers (equal to eight saltines); jalapeño-cheese spread; an airline-size packet of dry-roasted salted peanuts; presweetened, lemon-flavored instant-tea mix; powdered cocoa mix; a tiny bottle of Tabasco sauce; a package of M&M's; salt; an MRE heater pouch (more about this later); a tan plastic spoon (but no fork or knife); two pieces of green Chiclet-type chewing gum; a book of matches; a moist towelette; and a packet of toilet paper (22 sheets).

I heat up the beef stew, which looks like less-chunky Dinty Moore and—guess what—tastes like it too. Actually, it's not bad but awfully bland. What this baby needs is Tabasco. Ah, yes—perfect. Along with crumbled crackers, that makes it absolutely, uh, inoffensive. For a side dish, I squeeze some of the cheese spread, which is practically identical to Cheez Whiz, onto the bland, nearly salt-free cracker. I don't feel like having two beverages, so I just mix up the cocoa with hot water, and it's great. The peanuts and M&M's are the reward for cleaning my plate. One meal down, six to go.

Personally, I would have preferred more stew and fewer side dishes, but I'm not the target audience. "These meals are geared for a nineteen-year-old soldier running around all day carrying an eighty-pound pack and a rifle," says Jim Lecollier, a contracting officer with the Defense Supply Center, in Philadelphia, part of the Department of Defense. "They're nutritionally balanced and have about 1,300 calories per meal." The moist components, like the stew, are precooked; sealed in a pouch—sort of a flat bag—made of bonded layers of plastic, nylon, and aluminum foil; and heat-sterilized the same way canned goods are. This explains why most of the MRE entrées I tried tasted canned. Stored at 70 degrees, they can last for more than eight years (frightening thought), although the DOD keeps them for only three.

*Meal 2, breakfast.* The military does not offer breakfast-type MREs. Soldiers need protein and a lot of calories three times a day, but the thought of something like pork chow mein at seven in the morning is making me bilious. Luckily, my lunch package contains two Nature's Valley peanut-butter granola bars, crumbly and good. Yesterday's instant-tea mix is great hot; it doesn't even taste like instant. Somehow I feel guilty for enjoying this meager repast; maybe I should put on camouflage to eat this or dig a foxhole in the backyard.

Even though breakfast isn't offered, there is variety in the selection of regular entrées—24 choices, including 4 vegetarian ones. For a reality check, the Department of Defense conducts focus groups and taste tests. "We'll take some new entrées to, say, a base in Texas and ask the troops what they like," says Frank Johnson, a spokesman for the Defense Supply Center. Each year, the two least-popular meals are dropped and two new ones are added.

*Meal 3, lunch.* Bunch of wimps, that's what they are. Nobody in the *Texas Monthly* editorial department will so much as take a bite of my MRE. "Oh, no, that's fine," they say. "Er, I think I hear my mother calling." Are they clairvoyant? The cheese tortellini with tomato sauce is a dead ringer for something out of a Chef Boyardee can. Happily, a fresh bottle of Tabasco is at hand. The sauce manufacturer, the McIlhenny Company, of Louisiana, should get a medal of honor from the DOD. As for the rest, the applesauce is fine, but the peanut butter isn't salty enough. By the way, the toilet paper comes in handy for blowing your nose when it's running like a faucet after eating a meal drenched in Tabasco.

As I've opened each new pouch over the past day and a half, I've been struck by how reassured I feel when I pull out a brand-name product and how dubious I feel about the generic foods. Lecollier explains that the military makes a point of including major labels: "If you were a soldier out in the middle of nowhere, wouldn't it make you feel better to open up a package and find something that reminded you of home?"

*Meal 4, dinner.* I've conned my friend Robert into having

supper with me. We'll see whether he's still speaking to me after tonight. We are splurging and having the "grilled restructured chopped and formed" beefsteak and the cooked ham slice with "natural juices" and "smoke flavoring." Robert decides that they're actually edible sponges. I think they're more like a better class of Spam. The beef comes, oddly, with canned-tasting Mexican rice. The side dish for the ham is innocuous noodles in butter-flavored sauce. We split his hot cocoa and my lemon pound cake. He skips his two Tootsie Rolls. The cake isn't homemade quality, but relatively speaking, it's quite good. For once, I'm not tempted to add Tabasco.

The Wornick Company, the private business that makes and packages meal components under contract with the Department of Defense, has been turning out MREs for about twenty years (it also makes microwaveable entrées for 7-Eleven). At its branches in McAllen and Cincinnati, Wornick produced approximately 780,000 cases of MREs—twelve meals to a case—for the military last year, a fourth of the 3.1 million cases made nationwide. (The rest were made by companies in Indiana and South Carolina.) The DOD expects to buy 3.1 million cases of MREs again this year.

*Meal 5, breakfast.* Oh, groan. I guess it's presweetened tea and a granola bar again. I would kill for a latte.

*Meal 6, lunch.* Today is the day that I attempt to heat my meal—chicken with cavatelli (shell pasta)—with the chemical heater included in every pack. Since I nearly failed high school chemistry, the prospect of accidentally setting the office kitchen on fire is filling me with angst. After reading the instructions five times, I pour water into the special heater pouch, slip in the chicken with cavatelli (still in its package), fold the top over, and wait while—miracle of miracles—the promised water-activated chemical reaction occurs (don't ask me to explain it). The now-warm chicken patty looks like pressed meat but tastes okay. And the pasta with its tomatolike sauce is considerably better than yesterday's cheese tortellini; only half a tiny bottle of Tabasco is required to make it palatable. Today's drink is a cherry Kool-Aid-type beverage (a little weird with the tomato sauce, but my standards are eroding fast). Dessert is more pound cake, topped with good blackberry jam squeezed from a plastic pouch. My après-dinner beverage is Taster's Choice instant coffee. Skittles fruit-flavored candies stand in for chocolate truffles.

*Meal 7, dinner.* Oh happy day! *The West Wing* is on, and I'm having my last MRE, chili and macaroni, in front of the TV. The chili—which contains soy protein as well as ground meat—is not as bad as the ham slice but not as good as the beef stew (did I actually say the beef stew was good?). I've started measuring quality in TS units—the amount of the Tabasco sauce that's required to render a meal pleasantly palatable. The chili mac gets a 1—a whole bottle. Dessert is—please, not pound cake again. I know there are other desserts out there—fudge brownies and fig bars, to name two—but I didn't happen to get them.

What's my final take on surviving for 48 hours on MREs? I'm still alive (take that, Evan Smith). I didn't get indigestion. I gained half a pound. And I realized how much I take for granted certain things that are missing from these hardy combat-food packets, like a variety of vegetables and fruits. I also developed a profound appreciation for what our soldiers in the field endure, culinarily speaking. To them I raise a glass of presweetened, lemon-flavored instant tea and say, "God bless America."

*January 2002*

# CRITTERS AND FRITTERS

ANNE DINGUS

Vintage cookbooks are among my favorite heirlooms, although you might not want me to plan a meal with them. Barbecued armadillo, anyone?

WHEN IT COMES TO GOOD COOKING, I am the bad egg of the family. Many of my meals are unintentionally flambé, and I commit assorted chefly sins—for example, dumping flour directly from the bag into the bowl. (If my kids hadn't long ago borrowed the sifter for sandbox duty, it would be in mint condition today.) In short, my kitchen efforts are recipes for disaster. It's ironic, then, that I'm the one who inherited dozens of tattered old cookbooks from amateur chefs on both sides of the family.

Although I've never prepared a single dish from any of these lowbrow heirlooms, I can't bear to toss them out. I can pick out the best-loved recipes—not only because I've eaten the final results but also because the pages appear alarmingly blood-spattered and fly-specked. But as someone who often forgets to turn off the mixer before lifting the beaters out of the batter, I know what those spots really are: souvenirs of long-gone biscuits, pies, and casseroles. So I'm keeping these treasures—dog-ears, broken backs, and all. Someday, when my sons discover that their late mother collected dirty books, they can do the tossing for me.

Vintage Texas cookbooks are just a whole lot of fun. Even the earliest contain continental classics like chicken marengo and crêpes suzette—as if the nearest general store stocked white wine and curaçao alongside the calico and seed corn—as well as shuddery concoctions such as whey punch, liver-onion patties, and parsnip fritters. I love to flip through them and puzzle over forgotten words like "marlow" (fancy custard) and "Cottolene" (a shortening much favored in Texas because it came from cottonseed). A short sentence or two could mean a day's work: "Select a 4-weeks' old little pig. Clean and scald." Some cultural references completely escape me—one quote that launches a cookbook's pastry section reads "What a time the monster is cutting up the cake"—and the factual errors can crack me up. A confused homemaker clearly thought mangoes and muskmelons were the same fruit; an assertively Texan cookbook touts "Gov. Phelps' Egg Nog"—but we never had a Governor Phelps; and one beef-eater, obviously unfamiliar with Louisiana cuisine, donated a recipe for "filet gumbo." The stilted language provides more cheap laughs: for instance, "Dress the turkey yourself" (in a widdle hat and coat?) and the Hannibal Lecterish directive "Wash and trim one medium-sized heart." But the era had its blinders, and some things aren't funny. A recipe for a dessert combining "macaroons, nuts, and a 35¢ bottle of cherries" is labeled "Jew Pudding," and some troglodyte slopped together ground beef, spaghetti, mushrooms, and corn and dubbed the result "Dago's Delight."

There's another reason I love old cookbooks. Just as today's food literature—chichi, glossy, even lascivious—reflects modern life, so do the modest little volumes of yesteryear preserve the mundane details of a vanished society. The chief ingredients of cookbooks today are alluring photos and enticing words ("pomegranate salsa," "lemongrass-cream nage"). In the past, when books of any kind were precious and rare, a typical cooking guide was set in teeny type with few illustrations. It likely included—besides "receipts" for everything from oyster bisque to pecan brittle—medical advice, gardening tips, and mawkish homilies. Even back then, advertisements subsidized printing costs, and they are earnest if often bewildering. ("Dr. Hughes' Grape Baking Powder"? Please tell me it wasn't flavored.) Best of all are the household hints, dozens of which fill the back of most manuals. Here's an 1883 suggestion for sweeping a carpet: "Rub and wash four large

potatoes, put them in a chopping-bowl and chop into pieces the
size of a pea, sprinkle them over the floor, brush well over the carpet with your broom, then sweep thoroughly." Alas, there is no
subsequent tip titled "Cleaning Spud Schmutz From Rugs."

One of my favorite family hand-me-downs is the *Matagorda Cook Book*, a joint effort by that town's Methodist churchwomen 95 years ago. I spent part of every childhood summer in Matagorda with my maternal grandparents, he a dedicated hunter and fisherman who set out many Saturday mornings to catch or shoot dinner and she a renowned cook who jumped up to heat a skilletful of Crisco as soon as she heard him pull into the driveway. She was also game for whipping up any dessert, anytime (her dewberry cobbler!). Mimi, as I called her, was a cookbook junkie, though she frequently rejiggered recipes ("increase sugar to 2½ cups") and penciled commentary into the margins ("delicious toasted!"). She and the *Matagorda Cook Book* faithfully hewed to the same cooking commandments, the first of which might have been "For hot seafood dishes thou shalt ladle on the pork fat or the butter, and in cold ones spare not the mayonnaise." I'm also fond of Mimi's bilingual copy of *Memorial Book and Recipes*, issued in 1957 by the Czech Catholic Home for the Aged in tiny Hillje, near El Campo. It contains nine versions of kolaches, some of which are simply terrifying (no recipe should contain a sentence beginning "Next morning. . ."). Some of the hints, such as "Old felt hats make attractive hot pads for the table," would haunt Heloise.

On my father's side, Aunt Ina ruled the range. She had a food sense that was partly innate and partly acquired from decades spent assembling massive noon meals for the hands on the family farm. She could turn a fat, squawking hen into hot fried chicken in 45 minutes flat. I never saw Aunt Ina use a cookbook, but after she died, one surfaced among her things. It's a homemade paperback, dated 1966 and titled *Gressett Grub* (the Gressetts were her mother's clan). I value this booklet for its two shocking postchildhood revelations: First, blood relatives I loved and respected not only ate but baked fruitcake; and second, the foods in *Gressett Grub* are arranged by gastronomical merit: breads first, then desserts, then meats, and last (and least), the stepchild side dishes, more than half of which involve Jell-O. This culinary pecking order goes a long way toward explaining why I will never tip over in a high wind.

Some Texas cookbooks aren't amusing; they're laughable. I can really work up a hissy fit over *The Texas Cookbook* (1949), by Arthur and Bobbie Coleman. I don't know the Colemans, and I suspect by now they're tending that great Aga in the sky, but they thought reds and pintos were the same frijoles and even used the words "chiles" and "pimientos" interchangeably. Among their purportedly authentic Texan recipes are spiced eel, mutton curry, barbecued armadillo with sesame seeds, and stewed rattlesnake with shallots and red wine. But I was grateful to learn that, when I'm preparing to bake my freshly killed possum, I can soak the carcass in hot lye to remove the fur. Silly me—all this time I've just been skinning it with my bowie knife!

One despairs to think that this kind of hookery-cookery book survives while other legitimate gems are falling through the kitchen-floor cracks. Fortunately, the International Association of Culinary Professionals (IACP) is on the case. The group of some four thousand chefs, writers, restaurateurs, and the like held its annual meeting in Dallas in April. Along with the usual noshing and sloshing, the foodies enjoyed a special treat: the release of four vintage cookbooks, the first wave of an ambitious publication plan. Of the inaugural four, three are Texan: *The El Paso Cook Book*, compiled by the Ladies Auxiliary of that city's YMCA in 1898; *The Lone Star Cook Book*, sold by the Ladies of the Dallas Free Kindergarten and Training School in 1901; and *Mexican Cooking: The Flavor of the 20th Century—That Real Mexican Tang*, printed in San Antonio in 1911 for the Gebhardt Chili Powder Company.

Why would such an elite group decide to reissue a trio of obscure cooking manuals from a state that many nonresidents still regard with suspicion? After all, there are far-more-famous tomes out there. That's the point, says New Yorker Andrew F. Smith, who selected the titles; the IACP wants to save endangered treasures. "As far as I know, only three copies of *The Lone Star Cook Book* have survived," he says, "and there are only six known copies of *The El Paso Cook Book*." Smith is a food historian who has written or edited eighteen books, including last year's 1,584-page *Oxford Encyclopedia of Food and Drink in America*. He acknowledges that the choices were, in part, a tip of the toque to the association's host city, Big D, but also reveals that "Tex-Mex and Texas barbe-cue rank near the top of my personal culinary hierarchy." As for the Gebhardt pamphlet, which was originally hawked for 15 cents, Smith firmly IDs it as "the first Mexican American cookbook." Holy *mole*—that's like the Ark of the Covenant! Say *no más*.

Clearly, cookbooks in early Texas were few and far between, right? Wrong. At least 402 had been published by the end of 1936, Texas's centennial year. This factoid comes to us courtesy of Elizabeth Borst White, of Houston, a medical librarian and cookbook collector who has researched a bibliography of Texas's culinary works, starting in 1855, when Gail Borden (the milk man) put out an eight-page booklet explaining how to prepare his dry, slow-to-spoil "meat biscuit." White's labor of love, a special edition of which sold out at the IACP fest, led her to some long-shelved gems, such as the *K.K.K. Cook Book* (Honey Grove, 1894; the initials stood for Kute Kooking Klub) and *300 Ways to Please a Husband* (Lockhart, 1915). Fifty-one titles were advertising promo-tions, including the 1915 *Economy Cookbook* from Imperial Sugar, of Sugar Land, which called for the company's products in just about everything—not just candies and cakes but also vegetables (lima beans, pickled beets) and even one-dish meals like tuna lasagne and pot roast.

Which reminds me, it's dinnertime and I've got to get that possum in the oven. No lye.

*June 2005*

# STOCK TIPS

PATRICIA SHARPE

At the Texas Culinary Academy, in Austin, I chopped vegetables, roasted bones—and got a taste of what it's like to be a chef.

**AT SIX-TWENTY ON A TUESDAY MORNING LAST FALL,** jittery from too much coffee and not enough sleep, I stepped into a classroom kitchen at the Texas Culinary Academy, in Austin. Chef-instructor Gary Ackerman was directing half a dozen student volunteers who were hustling around preparing trays of ingredients for the class. Ackerman, 45, seemed to be doing about ten things at once. "Nice to have you here," he said, looking up from a cutting board. "Have a seat." Then he went back to chopping off carrot tops.

I found a chair at one of several long tables and put on my borrowed chef's jacket and toque. The large, high-ceilinged room—more than two thousand square feet—was filling up with the forty students who were taking the class. They straggled in, fumbling around for their recipes and helping one another tie their scarves ("This is the manly way; that's the girly way," someone said, indicating a Windsor knot and a granny knot). Everyone had on a white jacket, the traditional black-and-white-checked pants, and close-fitting white caps. (I got to wear a toque, which students are awarded when they graduate, because I was a guest.) Although most were in their twenties, a few looked like middle-aged career changers, with a 3 to 2 ratio of men to women. The

Patricia
Sharpe

majority were Anglo or Hispanic, with only one black student (the class had no Asian students, though they make up about 10 percent of the academy's overall enrollment). This diverse group included chef wannabes who had come from as far away as Michigan to gamble that they could parlay $36,000 into a lucrative job. I had come because I wanted to find out what it was like to train to be a chef these days. And, frankly, I wanted to see how I would perform under pressure: Would I rise to the occasion like a soufflé or collapse into a puddle of goo?

Although not the only professional cooking school in Texas, the Texas Culinary Academy (TCA) may well be the most ambitious and fastest growing. It started out in 1981 as a small-potatoes apprenticeship program called Le Chef but hit the big time two years ago when it moved into its present glitzy digs, a $9-million, 52,000-square-foot building in North Austin. Its recent rise to prominence is a testament, in part, to the shrewdness of its youthful director, Harvey Giblin, who at 35 bears more than a passing resemblance to Doogie Howser, M.D. While the state's other culinary schools—El Centro College, in Dallas; St. Philip's College of San Antonio; Del Mar College, in Corpus Christi; and the two highly regarded Art Institutes in Houston and Dallas— graduated a total of some 250 baby chefs in 2003, the TCA had 420 graduates (and an enrollment of 750 students). That number hardly compares with the 1,200 who graduated from the Harvard of cooking colleges, the Culinary Institute of America (CIA), in Hyde Park, New York, but then the academy hasn't been around for 32 years either.

Every six weeks, a new group of students arrives, keeping the academy's six kitchens—each of which cost around $350,000 to equip—humming for three five-hour shifts a day, five days a week. When they finish the program, the students will have survived twelve months of classes and kitchen practice plus a three-month paid "externship" in an actual restaurant; some of their predecessors have worked at Charlie Trotter's, in Chicago; Lupa, in New York (one of Mario Batali's restaurants); and the Food Network. Unless their parents are wealthy, they will have racked up loans totaling $36,000 for tuition and $2,000 for equipment and books (the CIA charges about $15,000 a year for its two-year program).

They will also wear battle scars from real knives and real flames and, if all has gone well, still have a burning desire to cook. Ninety-six percent of them will get jobs. Some of the best and brightest have ended up at restaurants including the Mansion on Turtle Creek, in Dallas, and Spago, in Los Angeles, as well as cruise ship dining rooms.

The TCA teaches French preparations and terms; in my class, we learned the definitions of "demi-glace" (a rich brown sauce reduced by half to a thick glaze) and "pincer" (to brown in fat before adding liquid). But the French focus alone is not unusual. What sets the TCA apart is its status as an affiliate of the historic Le Cordon Bleu, of Paris; it's one of eleven in the United States. Since Giblin forged an alliance with the crème de la crème of cooking colleges in 2002, the TCA has taught the Cordon Bleu curriculum, and representatives of the French academy drop by periodically for a little tête-à-tête and to see how things are going (which must be like knowing that the Michelin guidebook inspector is in your dining room prodding a lamb chop). Although French principles and recipes undergird the course of study, dishes from other nations are taught as well. Today we would learn how to make brown veal stock, one of the most fundamental preparations of classic French cooking. Feeling the way I do in a theater just before the curtain goes up, I dug out my notebook and a pen.

At exactly six-thirty, chef-instructor John Mims, 54, called the roll. "I have Band-Aids left over from yesterday," he announced, waving them in the air. "Not as many cuts as expected. Excellent." Then Ackerman, wearing the usual chef's jacket and a toque, stepped to the center of the room and faced the students, who were perched on chairs around stainless-steel tables arranged in a U-shape. Set out on more tables behind him were trays of veal knuckle bones, bins of whole carrots and onions, and bunches of celery. More trays held bay leaves, peppercorns, cloves, fresh flat-leaf parsley, and canned tomato paste. (There were also chicken carcasses for the chicken stock that we would prepare today as well, but it was decidedly subordinate to the brown veal stock.)

"Can anyone define the word 'stock'?" Ackerman asked.

"It's a clear, thin, flavorful liquid," somebody volunteered.

"Yes," Ackerman said. "What else?"

Patricia
Sharpe

No one responded, so he supplied the answer: "A stock is a thin, flavorful liquid that is derived from the cooking of bones or vegetables." We all scribbled away madly.

"Now," he continued, "what are the uses of stock?"

Several students suggested sauces and soups. Ackerman added consommés, plus braised or simmered dishes like galantines, fancy molded pâtés covered in aspic, a.k.a. jellied stock.

"In short," he said, punching out the words, "stock is *everywhere*. You have to be a stock *expert*. It is as important to a chef as his *knife*."

He paused dramatically for this to sink in.

Ackerman, whom we addressed as "Chef" or "Chef Gary," was a good teacher, patient but demanding. People who work in kitchens, under pressure, are infamous for their black humor, and he was no exception. Asking us to please not traipse through the area where he usually stood, he added, "Unless you're running for the door holding a bloody stump." Before he came to the TCA, he had been a chef and a caterer and had owned his own restaurant. His 25 years of experience are typical of the academy's faculty.

During his talk he covered the basics, explaining terms like "bouquet garni" (a mix of herbs such as thyme and parsley) and "sachet" (a little cheesecloth bag to hold spices and herbs like bay leaves, cloves, and peppercorns), pausing from time to time to demonstrate the steps for making a brown veal stock, absolute perfection always being the goal.

The procedure—in case you want to try this at home, kids—is as follows: First you brown some veal knuckle bones in a 375- or 400-degree oven for an hour, until they turn a dark brown. Meanwhile, prepare a mirepoix (named for, you guessed it, a Frenchman, Charles de Lévis, duc de Mirepoix). It consists of two parts roughly cut onion to one part each celery and carrot, and it makes the stock flavorful and aromatic.

You roast the mirepoix with the veal bones for fifteen minutes, then remove the pan from the oven and brush the bones with tomato paste (canned is used because it is high in acid and is made from ultra-ripe tomatoes). You put the bones and vegetables back in the oven until the paste has caramelized, about ten to fifteen more minutes, then toss everything into a stock pot filled with water (our class had two 24-gallon pots, each two feet tall).

After that, you pour yourself a glass of red wine (you deserve it). When you're sufficiently relaxed, add a bit of the wine and some hot water to the roasting pan to help dissolve the crusty, dark *fond* (meaning "foundation"). Then scrape the pan like mad and add those tidbits to the simmering stock-to-be. Finally, throw in a sachet and a bouquet garni. When students queried Acker- man about amounts—"How much tomato paste, Chef?"—he first explained what he was doing and why ("I want a thin layer, so it will dry out and start to caramelize") and then gave a measure- ment for the quantity of bones we were using. When someone was surprised that he didn't use measuring cups or spoons, he said, "Use your *judgment*. A recipe lets you cook one dish. A technique lets you cook anything."

Finally it was time for us to do what we had come to do: play with knives and fire and get into trouble. Two students invited me to help them, and we quickly found out how hard it is to keep everything straight when forty people are running around a huge kitchen calling out "Behind you!" as they barrel through on their way to and from the sinks and stoves carrying hot veal bones and greasy pans. Somehow we mistakenly set our oven at 325 degrees instead of 375, and after 45 minutes our veal bones were only a pitiful, pasty beige instead of a yummy brown. Then when our chicken stock boiled over, we turned the flame down so far that it blew out and the stock stopped cooking altogether for who knows how long.

Barely controlled chaos reigned: Every time you bent over to open the oven door, you would whack somebody with your rear end. Getting to a sink was like skiing the giant slalom at the Olympics. Mysterious forces caused tongs and knives to vanish when needed most. After an hour, I concluded that I personally could land a part in any sequel to *Dumb and Dumber*, but my partners did most things right and we finished on time, including helping wipe and sweep the whole kitchen. Our class's two communal pots of brown veal stock would simmer for eight to nine hours after we left. When we needed them two days later, they would be ready to go.

Patricia
Sharpe

On Thursday morning, Ackerman stood in the middle of the class with our veal stock in a pot beside him. He dipped a spoon into it. Voilà! In the intervening day our stock had been miraculously transformed into something rich and strange. Cooked down, strained, and chilled, it had morphed into a beautiful, translucent, solid golden-brown mass: veal Jell-O. He held up a quivering spoonful. "This is amazing stuff," he said. "You should be proud. Good work!" We basked in the praise. It was thrilling to witness the transformation of such mundane things—bones, vegetables, water—into something so refined.

As Ackerman continued and we got ready to make a series of eight sauces using our stock—demi-glace, *espagnole, chasseur,* Robert, and more—I thought about how the principles of a culinary education parallel the rules of stock-making: Start with good ingredients, learn the moves, and astonishing changes can happen. The five hours went by in a blur. Somehow our team of three managed to make our eight sauces in the time allotted, and when Ackerman came around to grade them, we got—on a twenty-point scale—eighteens, nineteens, and twenties. Eighteen meant the sauce had a couple of minor flaws; nineteen and twenty meant it was good enough to serve in a restaurant. We were so surprised we just stared at each other, grinning idiotically from ear to ear.

After class was over, I walked down the hall to the academy office and turned in my jacket and toque. Briefly, I thought about asking if I could keep the hat, even though it made my hair stand out like sprigs of parsley. I wasn't quite ready to give it back.

*January 2004*

# THE ART OF THE MEAL

PATRICIA SHARPE

After a hard morning of relishing Rothkos and viewing Van Goghs, take time out to appreciate a culinary masterpiece or two. Five of the state's best museums have cafes worthy of their collections, with menus ranging from the classic to the postmodern.

BACK IN THE OLDEN DAYS, art museums did not have restaurants. Why would anyone eat at a museum? That made about as much sense as taking a picture with a telephone. But modern life is all about changing paradigms, and museums now give as much thought to designing their dining rooms as to planning their galleries. When New York's Museum of Modern Art reopened in 2004 after an extensive makeover, its dining options got almost more press than its redo.

In Texas, the unwritten rule that forbade eating in the vicinity of great art was breached by the Kimbell Art Museum, in Fort Worth, in 1981. Soon, tourists and townies alike were crowding into its popular buffet. The tide had turned, and when it came time to add a new wing or building, museums began to allot serious space to feeding the hordes. "Refreshments will be served" became the mantra of any museum worth its Alexander Calder mobile.

What awaits the famished Texas art lover today? Happily, you can dine without leaving the air-conditioned comfort of the building at five art institutions in Dallas, Fort Worth, and Houston. Three other cities—Austin, El Paso, and San Antonio—lag behind, although the Blanton Museum of Art, in Austin, plans to catch up next spring. To size up the offerings, I traveled the state, eating Moroccan chicken salad in Fort Worth, veggie burgers in Houston, and tempura shrimp in Dallas. For those museums without cafes, I did a little off-site foraging, picking a favorite restaurant that was within walking distance or a short drive. Here's what's on the menu for your next cultural and gastronomical tour of Texas.

## DALLAS

### SEVENTEEN SEVENTEEN AND ATRIUM CAFE, DALLAS MUSEUM OF ART

If you have the money, honey, not to mention the time, the place to eat at the Dallas Museum of Art is Seventeen Seventeen. You might even need reservations, because it's popular with downtown power brokers in suits and ties and curator types in black clothes and arty eyewear. While a friend and I waited for our food, we conversed over blessedly subdued music and enjoyed the setting, a minimalist white room looking out onto a terrace and the city beyond. Chef Mike Dimas's daily specials run to the likes of mahimahi with red pepper—dill butter sauce, while his regular menu (which changes about four times a year) lists main courses such as a pecan-crusted chicken breast with a maple glaze and a pan-roasted tenderloin in a shallot demi-glace.

Our entrée salads were the perfect antidote to a blistering hot day. Mine was a mound of varied fresh lettuces served in a rice-paper basket, like an Asian tortilla bowl; the greens were adorned with four hefty, crisp-fried tempura shrimp in a sweetish Thai chile vinaigrette. I loved it. My friend ordered the monster Upside Down Cobb Salad. While the mixed greens were a little wet, that deficiency was balanced by a bounty of blue cheese, cooked egg, and mashed avocado, plus applewood-smoked bacon and cured salmon (alternative protein choices being ribeye or smoked chicken).

For dessert, we followed our unwavering rule: When panna
cotta is offered, you must accept. Chef Dimas's light, silky custard was infused with a shot of fresh lemon juice and surrounded
by a heap of blueberries. Not a bad reward for a pathetic lack of
willpower.

As for the museum's other venue, the Atrium Cafe, let me be
candid: This is where you eat if you're either in a hurry or have
done your parental duty by force-feeding culture to a bunch of
kids. It's inexpensive and fast, and it occupies a wonderful, soar-
ing space decked out with fantastic glass vessels by artist Dale
Chihuly. But as for the food—sandwiches, soups, salads, tacos,
desserts—the words "supermarket cafe" spring to mind. Enough
said. *1717 N. Harwood, 214-515-5179.*

## NASHER CAFE BY WOLFGANG PUCK, NASHER SCULPTURE CENTER

I dearly wanted Nasher Cafe's food to be great, because the little
dining room is so sleek and stylish. One entire wall is glass, giving
you a view of the garden and its amazing statuary, including Jona-
than Borofsky's vision of fiberglass people walking up a pole and
into the sky. The dining room is open and airy, with white freesias
on the tables. Even the Scandinavian-designed flatware is slick. So
imagine how disappointed my friend and I were when the interesting menu turned out to be decidedly flawed.

Oh, it wasn't all terrible. But it wasn't what it should have been
for a cafe operated by Wolfgang Puck Catering, a company that
runs museum restaurants around the country. And, actually, the
first dish we tried was excellent, a tangy, slightly chunky tomato
soup that tasted of bountiful summer gardens. It was lovely, but
after that, things went downhill.

At the clerk's suggestion—you order at a small, well-designed
counter—I got a ham-and-cheese panini. The alleged Spanish
serrano ham turned out to be the pinkest, most ordinary version
of that mahogany-hued meat I've ever seen, and the sandwich's
touted mustard aioli was undetectable to the eye or palate. As for
my friend's entrée, the crisp, golden-brown chicken breast looked

pretty and smelled divine, but the meat was tragically overcooked. We had hopes for the side dish of mashed potatoes, but while they tasted great, they were nearly as liquid as cream gravy. The last item on the plate was a precise arrangement of grilled asparagus spears, and I'm happy to report that they were delightful—all three of them.

By this time, we were fairly demoralized, so we decided to restore our good cheer by splitting a tarte Tatin. Being a foe of overly sweet desserts, I hate to say this, but it needed more sugar. On the plus side, though, we could really taste the apples, and the puff pastry was properly buttery and flaky. I'm not sure Wolfie would be proud, but at least he wouldn't be totally embarrassed to be associated with it. *2001 Flora at Harwood, 214-242-5110.*


FORT WORTH

### BUFFET AT THE KIMBELL, KIMBELL ART MUSEUM

Locals call it the lunch line, but that hardly does justice to the Kimbell's small but soul-satisfying array of soups, salads, and desserts. Yes, you do walk through the Buffet at the Kimbell's short cafeteria line. But you forget that mundane detail once you're seated in the long room with its high ceilings and creamy Italian marble walls. In a central atrium a few feet away, flower beds of pink caladiums surround sculptor Aristide Maillol's semi-reclining bronze nude (it always bothers me that the poor thing is teetering on one hip and looks as if she might fall off her pedestal at any minute).

The chef and manager of the dining room is 25-year veteran Shelby Schafer, and of all the dishes she does, soups are my favorite. If the chilled guacamole soup is offered the day you visit, get a mugful; it's as tart and pungent as gazpacho. In fact, if the hearty chicken, sausage, and mushroom combo is also on the menu, have two soups. I could eat that one winter or summer, rain or shine.

Proceeding on down the line, you should definitely help yourself to the old-fashioned curried chicken salad. Another quaint option is the quiche, though this one is actually modern, with basil pesto stirred into a feta- and cheddar-enriched custard. By THE ART OF comparison, the smoked-turkey sandwich seems perfunctory, THE MEAL even with multigrain bread.

By this time, you've come to the dessert lineup, which when we visited consisted of two cakes and a cherry-pecan brownie. The one we liked best was the plain, granny-worthy yellow cake, oddly called an Italian cream cake. If you typically skip dessert at noon and you happen to be in town on a Friday evening, come back for coffee and a sweet (or for dinner, offered once a week). A jazzy guitar-and-bass duo played when I was there, making a nice conclusion to a busy week. *3333 Camp Bowie Blvd., 817-332-8451.*

## CAFE MODERN, MODERN ART MUSEUM

I always have great conversations at Cafe Modern, and I'm convinced it has something to do with the setting: glass walls wrapping around a smart but comfy dining room; a shallow, Zenish lake outside; and the monumental museum building itself reflected in the shimmering water. Makes the mind relax, or expand, or something. Whatever the secret, the cafe is popular, bringing in residents and museumgoers alike. Chef Dena Peterson's food always sounds interesting and is often made with locally grown ingredients. On top of that, the prices are manageable; it's hard to pay more than $15 for an entrée and sides at lunch.

Speaking of conversations, I heard all about a colleague's French river-barge trip while I devoured a fantastically flavorful curried Moroccan chicken breast crusted in pistachios. It was served chilled on romaine lettuce with feta and a light lemon vinaigrette, and it was so good that I could readily believe that customers won't let Peterson take it off the menu. But while my entrée was flawless, my friend's squash blossom quesadilla was not: Barely lukewarm, it was also apparently devoid of squash blossoms (the waiter said there were mounds of the little cuties in the kitchen, but we deconstructed her entrée and could find nary a one).

The next evening (the dining room does dinner one Friday a month) I lucked out again with a perfectly cooked filet mignon in a satiny demi-glace bolstered with—are you ready?—Dr Pepper.

*Patricia
Sharpe*

Don't cringe; it's like adding port to a demi. On this visit, another globe-hopping friend made me green with envy by rattling on about her forthcoming trip to Turkey. (If you must know, I thought it was a little bit tacky that neither one of them wanted to hear about my fabulous trip to West Texas.) That night, she got the only truly disappointing dish we sampled: sadly overcooked braised duck accompanied by cannonball-like cornmeal-bacon dumplings. But we had no problems with our desserts. Her Ultimate Banana Pudding came in a martini glass with buttered rum sauce and toasted pound cake croutons, and I was completely happy with my great, soupy rhubarb-berry crumble under a crisp topping that reminded me of granola. *3200 Darnell, 817-840-2157.*

## HOUSTON

### CAFE EXPRESS, MUSEUM OF FINE ARTS, HOUSTON

What is this, the ticket queue for some Egyptian mummy blockbuster? There are two lines with twenty or more people in each one, and we're standing here starving. Move it, you all! Cafe Express, which runs the food concession for the Museum of Fine Arts, Houston, is hardly la-di-da, but then, it isn't trying to be. A Houston-based chain with additional locations in Dallas and Fort Worth, it occupies the middle ground between "fast" and "nice": You order at a counter and are issued a pager, which has a conniption fit when your food is ready.

The large, casual space on the lower level is functional but well designed, with arty faux palm trees and brightly colored tables. I quite like the menu's wide range of generous salads, sandwiches, soups, and pastas and its handful of entrées. And I absolutely adore the condiment bar in the middle of the room, where you can load up your lunch with scandalous amounts of imported olives, grated Parmesan, Italian peppers, red-wine vinegar, croutons, capers, jalapeños, pickled sun-dried tomatoes, bread sticks, fresh basil, and more.

Although my friend and I could have ordered a substantial main course, like grilled Mediterranean salmon with roasted artichoke hearts, we decided to go light. The veggie burger proved to be the typical patty on a bun, all right but nothing fabulous, along with varied fresh fruit. The Greek salad was a considerable step up, with romaine and plenty of feta cheese, kalamata olives, red onions, and sliced grilled chicken. From the condiment bar, I poured on about a gallon of lemon-flavored olive oil, no doubt causing a major profit loss for the day.

We considered indulging in bread pudding for dessert but decided instead to split a peanut butter cookie, which was good but not destined for greatness. As we were leaving, I noticed a separate order counter for box lunches. Next time, I'm getting one, and a glass of wine, and heading over to the museum's sculpture garden for my own personal picnic under a tree. *Audrey Jones Beck Building, 5601 Main, 713-639-7370.*

## FIVE MINUTES AWAY

Dining has not come to all of the major museums in the state, but good eats are within an easy walk or drive.

### AUSTIN

#### Near the Austin Museum of Art

Although Cibo, half a block away, is one of Austin's better Italian restaurants, for greater variety and good prices, you should walk two and a half blocks to **Louie's 106,** a business lunchers' haven with burnished wood paneling and marble floors. It offers an excellent rotisserie chicken plate with mashed potatoes and garlicky sautéed spinach, and the mussels dijonnaise have few peers. *106 E. Sixth, 512-476-2010.*

#### Near the Blanton Museum of Art

With its attractive rough-limestone walls, the **Clay Pit** looks like the old mercantile store it once was. Besides the affordable Indian lunch buffet, there are specialties like khuroos-e-tursh, chicken breast rolled around spinach in a cashew-almond cream sauce. Tip: The restaurant is about half a mile away, and if you walk south along Congress Avenue from Martin Luther King Jr. Bou-

levard, you can enjoy a view of Texas's majestic state capitol. *1601
Guadalupe, 512-322-5131.*

EL PASO

### Near the El Paso Museum of Art

A block and a half away is **Cafe Central,** arguably the city's most
elite dining spot. Here movers, shakers, and social mavens mingle
in an elegant cream-and-black room filled with original art. The
green-chile cream soup is a classic, and you will need extra sour-
dough bread to mop up the savory juices of the clams steamed in
Dos Equis beer. *109 N. Oregon, 915-545-2233.*

FORT WORTH

### Near the Amon Carter Museum

The Amon Carter is temporarily closed for repairs, but when it
reopens around the middle of August, you can take a break from
the art by driving to **Gloria's,** less than a mile away, for suste-
nance (and of course, you can always eat at the nearby Modern or
Kimbell). Part of a local chain offering Salvadoran and Mexican
cuisine, this upscale edition has lipstick-red walls and sidewalk
seating. Try the pupusas—chunky, pocketlike tortillas stuffed
with pork, cheese, or both. *Montgomery Plaza, 2600 W. Seventh,
817-332-8800.*

HOUSTON

### Near the Contemporary Arts Museum, Houston

The simplest solution is to eat at the nearby Museum of Fine Arts,
Houston, but it's an adventure to stroll to the **Tart Cafe,** located
less than half a mile away in a modern building that houses con-
temporary art galleries. The counter-order menu offers all tarts
all the time—plus a few salads and sandwiches—served up in
a casual, tall room with nine concrete-topped tables, black ban-

quettes, and zoomy-looking white vinyl chairs. *4411 Montrose Blvd., 713-526-8278.*

### Near the Menil Collection

Tucked into a convivial if sometimes cacophonous cottage less than half a mile away is **Da Marco,** the best Italian restaurant in the city. Specialties have included Chianti-braised short ribs and risotto laced with Norcia truffles (the black diamonds of truffledom). *1520 Westheimer Rd., 713-807-8857.*

## SAN ANTONIO

### Near the McNay Art Museum

Drive, we said, four fifths of a mile to **Silo Elevated Cuisine,** a relaxed but refined cafe in a converted older building (the entrance is at the rear, upstairs). Do not refuse come-ons for the chicken-fried oysters with mustard hollandaise or the seared sea scallops with saffron beurre blanc. Resistance is futile. *1133 Austin Hwy., 210-824-8686.*

### Near the San Antonio Museum of Art

The museum has a snack bar but not a restaurant. Luckily, **Liberty Bar** is just a mile away, so head for this stupendously quirky hot spot for sophisticated but homey cuisine. The appetizer of goat cheese in a lush sauce of morita chiles and Mexican raw sugar can make grown men weep, and regular customers salute the trinity of God, Mother, and Virginia Green's Chocolate Cake. *328 E. Josephine, 210-227-1187.*

*July 2007*

# SIGNATURE TEXAS FOODS

# ¡VIVA TEQUILA!

### PATRICIA SHARPE

It's still a hot shot and the coolest ingredients of a margarita. But in kitchens and bars across Texas, Mexico's favorite drink has a newfound respectability.

ONCE UPON A TIME, tequila had a serious image problem. Synonymous with boozy cantinas and monumental hangovers, it was the beverage of choice for fraternity debauches. Barmaids toted it around in holsters for customers to slug down in bizarre shooter rituals. And, of course, the song to which Pee Wee Herman did his memorable dance in *Pee Wee's Big Adventure* was—yes—"Tequila."

But today, all that has changed. The baby boom generation, always on the prowl for something different, has finally turned its attention from wine, single-malt Scotch, fine vodka, and gourmet beer to tequila. During the past twenty years, while the sales of almost all other liquors have declined, in some cases drastically, tequila has been the fastest-growing category of spirits in the country, more than doubling its market share. In 1994 alone, sales of the best brands, those the liquor industry calls the superpremiums, increased by 20 percent. Tequila it seems has turned into a class act. Bars now list it along with brandies and liqueurs for $5 and $6 a glass. Package stores sell the top labels for $35 to $40. Connoisseurs of wines and fine spirits order tequila straight, in snifters—the better to savor every nuance. And cooks are finding

Patricia
Sharpe

that it has a marvelous affinity for food, as both an ingredient and an accompaniment.

With appreciation has come a debunking of tequila myths: It is not cactus juice or Mexican moonshine; it does not make you hallucinate; it does not have a worm in the bottle. The truth is that tequila is as complex and subtle as cognac or eau-de-vie, that the best ones are aged in oak barrels like fine wines and whiskeys, and that it doesn't take years of study or an arcane vocabulary to appreciate its full-bodied, salty, smoky taste. All it takes is a trip to a reasonably well-stocked liquor store—and the company of a few friends who share your spirit of adventure.

## DEFINING IT

There's more to tequila than just clear and gold. In fact, there are four categories defined by Mexico's tequila law, the Norma Oficial Mexicana "Tequila." First enacted in 1949, the NOM does for tequila what the Appellation d'Origine Contrôlée does for French wines and cognac: It sets forth which plants may be used to make tequila and where they may be grown, and it spells out government-enforced manufacturing standards.

By law, tequila (which means "volcano" in Nahuatl, the Aztec language, and also refers to a vanished Indian tribe that once inhabited the area) is a double-distilled liquor made in Mexico from the fermented juice extracted from the heart of the blue agave plant: *Agave tequilana* Weber, "blue" variety. Of course, there's tequila and there's *tequila*. Pure tequila is always labeled 100 percent agave; everything else is blended, legally, with as much as 49 percent cane or other sugar before fermentation. Blended tequilas can taste just fine, but they lack the full flavor of the pure agave ones.

The following four categories can be either pure or blended.

Silver (*plata*) tequila, also known as white (*blanco*), is fresh from the still and crystal clear. It is not aged, although some producers give it a little "rest" in stainless steel tanks or oak barrels for up to 45 days. It may be bottled in Mexico, but more frequently it is shipped to the United States in tanker trucks or railroad cars and then bottled here. Silver tequila has the reputation of being harsh, and some is, but a well-made silver tequila from 100 percent blue agave can be excellent.

Gold tequila is, essentially, a creation for the American marketplace; the Spanish word *oro* is rarely used in Mexico. The legal designation is *joven abocado* ("youthful but mellowed"), and most gold tequila is actually silver tequila with caramel coloring added to impart a rich hue. Unfortunately, novice buyers often mistake gold tequila for either *reposado* or *añejo* tequila, two very different types.

*Reposado,* or "rested," tequila is briefly aged in oak between two months and one year, a process that takes the edge off the rambunctious young silver tequila. It may absorb a light straw color from the oak, or coloring may be added. Either way, *reposados* are quite popular in Mexico. Some fanciers think they are the best tequilas; others hold that the "repose" does little to enhance the flavor. Many *reposados* are 100 percent agave.

*Añejo,* or "aged," tequilas are the finest and most expensive, kept in oak barrels for at least one year (the word *añejo* comes from *año,* or "year"). Ideally, the aging balances the natural sweetness of the agave sugar and the astringent, tannic quality of the oak. *Añejos* take on a natural amber tone from the barrel— usually old whiskey barrels bought from U.S. distilleries. Most are 100 percent agave.

Unlike wine, tequila does not improve but rather goes "off" if barrel-aged for more than about four years; nor does it age in the bottle. And there are no tequila vintage years, because tequila is harvested year-round and the quality of the crop is consistent.

## TASTING IT

The best way to get to know tequila is to drink it, and the best way to do that is to throw a tequila tasting.

Limit your tasting to six varieties; more than that and it will be hard to keep them straight. Serving them in classic tulip-shaped wine glasses will concentrate the aroma, which is part of the pleasure. (If you use shot glasses, people will start slamming them down, and there goes your sophisticated atmosphere.) Give

your guests pencil and paper so they can make notes on their fa-
vorites. The point is to sip and savor, discuss and compare.

Have plenty of food to eat before and after the tasting—chips,
salsa, guacamole, fresh corn tortillas—but don't have anything too
salty. To clear your palate, drink cool water and eat some bread or
tortillas between samples.

In selecting the brands, try for a range of qualities. To es-
tablish a benchmark, you might start with the best-selling Jose
Cuervo silver. After that, to taste the difference between pure and
blended silvers, sample Herradura silver, a 100 percent agave tequila prized by connoisseurs. Your third brand might be Sauza
Conmemorativo, which is not 100 percent agave but is aged in oak
to a notable smoothness. For your last choices, concentrate on
añejos. Number four could be El Tesoro añejo; like Juan Valdés's
coffee beans, El Tesoro's agaves are harvested at perfect ripeness.
Your final selections could be Centinela and Patrón, two other excellent and deep-flavored brands.

One final tip: The tequila market has its own odd vocabulary.
"Premium" ($20 to $30) means good and "superpremium" ($35
to $40) means excellent. Unfortunately, a few undistinguished
brands fetch even higher prices; so called "ultrapremium" cost a
bundle, but the tequila inside the fancy bottles isn't necessarily superior. Better keys to quality are "Made in Mexico" and "100 percent agave" on the label.

### RATING IT

#### WHICH TEQUILA DO CONNOISSEURS DRINK?

Considering the nationwide popularity of Southwestern and
Mexican cooking, we figured the cuisine's leading chefs and restaurateurs might know a thing or two about tequila. So we placed
a call to the following people: Robert Del Grande of Cafe Annie and Arnaldo Richards of Pico's, Houston; Dean Fearing of
the Mansion on Turtle Creek and Stephan Pyles of Star Canyon,
Dallas; Mark Miller of Coyote Cafe and Miguel Ravago of Fonda
San Miguel, Austin; Jay McCarthy of Cascabel and Rick Gonzalez of El Mirador, San Antonio; Mick Lynch of Cafe Central in El

Paso; and Grady Spears of Reata, Alpine. (We also asked Bruce Auden of San Antonio's Biga, who confessed that he doesn't drink tequila.) Most of those polled specified the mellower *añejo* or *reposado* in their favorite brands.

The winners in the tequila sweepstakes were (drum roll, please): First place, Herradura, with seven votes. Second, Patròn, with six. Third, El Tesoro, with five. Chinaco—once the hardest tequila to find, because production was unpredictable, but soon to be available again—got three votes, and Centinela and Sauza Tres Generaciones got two each. After that, the scoring evened out with Jose Cuervo gold, Dos Reales, Porfidio, and several other Sauza products (Conmemorativo and Hornitos) netting a vote apiece.

## MAKING IT

The long, spiky leaves of the blue agave plant look like a freeze-frame explosion; an entire field of agaves is a series of starbursts arranged in tidy rows from roadside to horizon. Despite their needlelike tips, the 250 to 300 species of agave are not cacti but rather members of the lily family, relatives of yucca, amaryllis, and sansevieria. A blue agave blooms just once, eight to ten years after it takes root, and then it dies. If it is harvested too soon, it will be unripe. If it is harvested too late, the heart will have formed its once-in-a-lifetime bloom stalk and will be no good for making tequila. Timing is everything. Moving gingerly among these plants, workers known as *jimadores* ("harvesters") carry long-handled tools with spatulate chopping blades called *coas*. Spotting a suitable plant, the *jimador* shears off a few base leaves and uproots the plant with his foot. With rapid, precise strokes, he then slices off the remaining leaves. The end product is a fifty-to-one-hundred-pound green globe that strikingly resembles a pineapple and is, in fact, called a *piña*. After they are cut, the *piñas* are loaded onto donkeys or tossed into trucks and delivered to the distillery, where they begin their metamorphosis into tequila.

It used to be that all tequila distilling was a primitive, labor-intensive operation. And indeed, some distilleries, including the modern giants, Jose Cuervo and Sauza, still cook the *piñas* in

Patricia
Sharpe traditional stone-walled ovens for as long as 36 hours, followed by more hours of cooling. Yet other larger distilleries are highly mechanized: They use autoclaves—essentially giant pressure cookers—that steam the *piñas* rapidly. Here, as in other aspects of tequila making, the traditional distilleries claim to make a superior product, drawing an analogy between a spaghetti sauce that takes thirty minutes to make and one that is slowly simmered for hours. Others say that either method can be effective in experienced hands.

Before a *piña* is cooked, it has the smooth, firm texture of a turnip or jicama and a slightly bitter, herbal taste. Once it has been baked, it is surprisingly like a sweet potato in color, flavor, and consistency. All its starches have turned to sugar, transforming the vegetable into a strange, fibrous candy.

The next step is to extract the juice. Newer distilleries crush the *piñas* with modern machinery; a few older ones use a large circular stone called a *tahona*. Once crushed, the *piñas* are repeatedly washed with water to separate the juice from the fibers, and the resulting liquid is transferred to fermentation containers, either huge stainless steel vats (in the modern plants) or small wooden ones. Sugar syrups may be added at this stage if the tequila is to be a blend. The next ingredient is yeast, commercial or wild; the type influences the style or taste of the finished product. As fermentation proceeds, the brown beery liquid simmers and roils. At the end of the process, which can take a few hours to a few days, the sugars have been converted into a mild alcohol—not yet tequila, but getting closer.

The missing step is distillation, which can take place in traditional copper stills or stainless steel ones. The fermented brew is heated to boiling, and the resulting vapors are condensed to a clear liquid of about 40 proof. The "heads" and "tails"—alcohols produced during the first and last stages of the process—are discarded because they contain harsh, even toxic impurities. Then the "heart" of the distillate is piped into a second group of stills to be finished.

The crystal-clear alcohol that comes out of the still is, finally, tequila. At 110 proof or higher, it is strong stuff, which is why distilled water is added to dilute it to 80 proof. If it is to be aged, it is transferred to oak barrels; if not, it is bottled (in either Mexico or the United States) and ready to be sold.

## EXPLAINING IT

Confusion reigns, at least among *norteamericanos*, over the differences among pulque, mescal, and tequila. Many people think that the first two are primitive or semi-finished stages of the third (tequila *interruptus*, so to speak). This rowdy, rotgut image persists even though pulque and mescal are quite distinct and can be good, bad, or indifferent.

Pulque (pronounced "*pool*-keh") has the most ancient lineage, having been consumed in Mexico for more than two thousand years. Rich in nutrients, it was prized by the Aztecs, who reserved it for the aged and infirm as well as for nobles, warriors, and nursing mothers. Anyone else caught sneaking a drink could be sentenced to death. Until the twentieth century, pulque occupied an honored place as the drink of revolutionaries, artists, and great landowners. Today it is regarded as the solace of poor folk. In the rest of society, Tecate and Coca-Cola have taken its place.

Like tequila, pulque is made from the juice of agave plants (but not *Agave tequilana* Weber, "blue" variety). Unlike tequila, it is extracted from living plants instead of those that have been harvested and cooked, and it is fermented but not distilled. To put it politely, pulque is an acquired taste. White, foamy, and thick, with an alcoholic content of between 4 and 6 percent, it has an herbaceous or a vegetable flavor that is simultaneously acrid, sweet, and salty. Because it doesn't take well to bottling or storage, it must be consumed fresh and in the vicinity of where it is produced—primarily Mexico's Central Plateau.

Compared with pulque, mescal ("mes-*cahl*") is a youngster, a mere four centuries old at best. When the Spanish colonized Mexico in the sixteenth century, they brought with them the ancient art of distilling. They soon applied that art to the agave, a plant with proven potential for alcohol production.

The making of mescal is almost identical to the making of tequila; and, indeed, tequila was once called *vino mescal* or "mescal wine," reflecting the fact that it is essentially a highly refined mescal. The main differences are that the two liquors use different species of agave plants and that mescal is distilled once rather than twice. The Mexican government does not regulate mescal production, so the quality varies. Some mescals are subtle and complex; most are not. To smooth the harsh, typically smoky flavor, fruits and spices such as lime, prickly pear, pineapple, almonds, and cinnamon are frequently added.

Mexicans regard mescal as a tonic, a diuretic, a digestive aid, and an aphrodisiac, and they consume almost all the mescal that is made, though a few American bars are starting to stock it. In short, mescal is what tequila was twenty years ago; a drink for the daring. But given America's enthusiastic adoption of Mexico's music, dance, and food, we may be seeing a lot more of it soon.

### DRINKING IT

*ALTHOUGH A MARGARITA CONTAINS SIMPLE INGREDIENTS, A GOOD MARGARITA IS ANYTHING BUT SIMPLE.*

Your best choice for tequila is silver. It has a fresh, bright taste, and it lets the shimmering, light green color of the lime juice shine through. Gold tequila is a good second choice; if you're used to a slightly sweeter flavor, you may even prefer it. Either way, 100 percent agave tequila provides the most intense flavor. The choice of brand is up to you, but buy a decent one. On the other hand, don't use an expensive aged tequila in a margarita. Would you cook with Château Lafite-Rothschild?

Triple sec is the generic name for any triple-distilled clear liqueur produced from the skins of curaçao and other oranges. Read the label to find one that is made with natural, not artificial, flavorings. Better yet, buy Cointreau, the most famous and exotic triple sec. Grand Marnier—orange liqueur blended with cognac—is touted as the connoisseur's choice, but too much of it can overwhelm a margarita.

Ironically, the most important ingredient is often the hardest one to get: good lime juice. When they are in season, use sweet little round Mexican limes (Key limes are the same thing). Big, dark green Persian limes can be bought year-round, but they are often sour and thinly flavored. If you do use them, bolster their sweetness with a dash of simple syrup (see any general cookbook).

Now for the recipe. Everyone has a favorite, but in case you don't, try this Mexican version, which produces a margarita that is a little less sweet than most American ones:

1 ½ ounces silver tequila
½ ounce Cointreau
¾ ounce fresh Mexican lime juice

Before serving, run a lime wedge around the lip of a pretty, flared stemware glass and twirl the outer edge lightly in a saucer of kosher salt. Shake the drink with ice (preferably smallish cubes) and either strain it or serve it with the ice.

What about frozen margaritas? Don't even think of making one. You are a grown-up.

DEBATING IT

Who created the margarita, and when? It would be easier to identify the missing link between man and ape. So many margarita candidates have been put forward and so little hard evidence has been offered that the origin of the now-ubiquitous drink will probably never be known.

The most frequently told version is that the margarita was first made in the forties by an unnamed bartender in Palm Springs, California, to mimic—but soften—the classic combination of a shot of tequila accompanied by a lick of salt and a bite of lime.

A favorite story among Texans is that a bartender named Pancho Morales invented the margarita on July 4, 1942, at a Juárez bar named Tommy's Place ("The Man Who Invented the Margarita," *Texas Monthly*, October 1974). Supposedly, it all began when a woman requested a Magnolia (brandy, Cointreau, and an egg yolk topped with champagne). Morales was a little fuzzy on the recipe, so he improvised—and his ersatz creation was a big hit.

Another popular theory cites society hostess Margarita Sames

*Patricia*
*Sharpe*

(formerly of Dallas, now of San Antonio), who claims to have concocted the drink for Christmas houseguests at her Acapulco hacienda in 1948 ("Barroom Brawl," *Texas Monthly*, July 1991).

But of all the people said to be associated with the margarita, the one who deserves the most credit is Vern Underwood, who first imported Jose Cuervo tequila into the U.S. in 1945 and promulgated a great advertising slogan: "Margarita: It's more than a girl's name."

EATING IT

Tequila will always be a party drink, but it is also surprisingly versatile. Not only can you drink it before, during, and after a meal, but you can also cook with it: It blends wonderfully with chiles, garlic, onions, salsas, and Mexican *moles*; it mellows the sourness of citrus juices; and it has a natural affinity for nuts and seeds. A discreet splash even adds verve to desserts.

Irrepressible Austinite Lucinda Hutson chronicles her travels through tequila country in *¡Tequila! Cooking with the Spirit of Mexico* (Ten Speed Press, 1995), a chatty volume of tequila lore and some 135 Southwestern-oriented recipes, including this one for gazpacho macho.

> 4 large tomatoes, seeded and chopped
> 1 yellow bell pepper, seeded and diced
> 1 red bell pepper, seeded and diced
> 3 cloves garlic, minced
> 2 to 4 serrano chiles, seeded and minced
> 2 cucumbers, peeled, seeded, and diced
> 4 green onions, diced
> 1 medium white onion, diced
> ¼ teaspoon whole allspice
> ½ teaspoon whole black peppercorns
> ½ teaspoon whole coriander seeds
> 3 cups tomato juice
> 3 tablespoons fresh lime juice
> 1 cup good silver tequila

3 tablespoons sherry vinegar
3 tablespoons red wine vinegar
4 tablespoons olive oil
1 teaspoon salt
2 tablespoons chopped fresh cilantro
3 tablespoons chopped fresh basil

Put diced vegetables in a large bowl. Grind spices and add to vegetables along with liquids and salt, whisking in olive oil last. Chill at least 6 hours.

Before serving, stir in cilantro and basil. Serve with condiments—chopped avocado, boiled shrimp, chopped cilantro, croutons. Makes about 10 cups.

Some forty up-to-date Mexican recipes and a smattering of tequila facts make up Californians Ann and Larry Walker's *Tequila: The Book* (Chronicle Books, 1994), from which this recipe for drunken shrimp is taken.

24 large shrimp (about 2 pounds), peeled and deveined
2 tablespoons good silver tequila
1 tablespoon olive oil
1 tablespoon Worcestershire sauce
3 cloves garlic
1 teaspoon crumbled dried oregano
1 teaspoon salt
1 tablespoon paprika
1 fresh serrano chile, stemmed and seeded
½ cup fresh cilantro
oil for cooking

Put shrimp in a nonreactive bowl. Purée other ingredients in a blender and thoroughly toss with shrimp. Cover and refrigerate 1 hour. Cook shrimp with marinade over high heat, tossing, until shrimp turn bright pink, 1 to 2 minutes. Serves 6.

In this recipe for fiesta frijoles from *¡Tequila!*, you can arrange the corn as a golden ring instead of mixing it with the black beans. If you can't find chile-flavored tequila, simply and ¼ to ½ teaspoon of crushed dried red pepper to the tequila.

## For the marinade:

4 cloves garlic, minced
1½ teaspoons cumin seeds, toasted and coarsely ground
2 teaspoons dried oregano
3 tablespoons chile-pepper-flavored tequila
4 tablespoons red wine vinegar
2 bay leaves, preferably fresh, crushed
½ teaspoon salt
5 tablespoons olive oil

## For the bean mixture:

3½ cups cooked black beans, chilled and drained
4 serranos or jalapeños (or more, to taste), chopped
6 green onions with some of the green tops, chopped
1 cup chopped red onion
½ cup chopped fresh cilantro
2 tablespoons chopped fresh epazote (optional)
2 cups fresh sweet corn kernels, cold-tossed
6 Roma tomatoes, chopped, lightly salted, and drained in a
    colander
juice of 1 to 2 fresh limes
salt to taste

In a small bowl, combine all marinade ingredients except olive oil, then slowly whisk in the oil.

In a large bowl, combine all bean-mixture ingredients except lime juice and salt, then toss with marinade. Chill for several hours or overnight, stirring occasionally. (If the recipe is to be held overnight, add corn and tomatoes a few hours before serving.) Drizzle with fresh lime juice and add salt to taste before serving.

*August 1995*

# ROUND AND ROUND

PATRICIA SHARPE

Tortillas have been with us since the heyday of the Maya and the Aztecs. Now these simple small cakes are big business—but some are still made the old-fashioned way.

WHO KNOWS WHEN TORTILLAS WERE INVENTED, if "invent" is even the right word? The ancient Maya were mad about them: According to their mythology, the first tortilla was made by a Maya peasant as a gift to his king some 12,000 years ago. The Aztecs too had tortilla technology down flat, judging from observations recorded by a Spaniard named Francisco Hernández in 1651: "They make with the palms of their hands thin tortillas of medium circumference . . . Some make these breads a palm long, and four fingers thick, mixed with beans and roast them on a *comal*. But for the important Indians they prepare tortillas of sifted maize, so thin and clean they are almost translucent and like paper." The Spanish, knowing a good thing when they tasted it, did not tamper with this edible art form. Instead they embraced it, replacing the unpronounceable Aztec term *tlaxcalli* with the diminutive form of their own word for "cake," *torta*; hence, "tortilla" means "small cake." Over the intervening centuries, these delicious small cakes have flourished throughout the country of their origin (of which Texas, of course, was once part). Now they are commanding a larger stage.

Consider the following: Last year tortilla sales in the United

States totaled an estimated $4 billion, nearly three times as much as ten years ago; Americans consumed approximately 91 billion flour and corn tortillas (and this doesn't include chips). Tortillas are the fastest-growing segment of the U.S. baking industry, and they have become the most popular ethnic bread in the country, surpassing such wimpy contenders as bagels, naan, pita, and English muffins. Flour tortillas (which were invented after the Spanish brought wheat and lard to the New World) have surged in popularity following the creation of the wrap and now come in a multitude of flavors, including yummy ones like chile and spinach and dubious ones like blueberry and honey-apple-cinnamon. In short, these circular wonders are going where no tortilla has gone before: In 1999 industry giant Mission Foods even opened a tortilla plant in Coventry, England.

And yet these are also challenging times for tortillas, as the touchstones of the modern world—mechanization, modernization, and mergers—change how they are made and who makes them: What was once a cottage industry is fast becoming a global one. Check out most Texas supermarkets and you'll find the shelves dominated by national brands, including Mission (based in Irving and the biggest tortilla maker in the country), Guerrero (also made by Mission), and Fort Worth–based Tia Rosa. (All three labels, incidentally, are owned by subsidiaries of huge tortilla companies headquartered in Mexico.) Big supermarket chains like Fiesta and H-E-B even have their own labels and also carry some of the larger regional brands. The best way to patronize a local company, however, is to get in your car and make the trip to a real live tortilla factory, such as Austin's El Milagro or Houston's La Poblana, in a Hispanic neighborhood.

The smaller factories are dwindling—some that use their own name are really owned by the big companies—but they can still be found. One of the real old-timers is a place with an appropriately old-fashioned name, the Sanitary Tortilla Manufacturing Corporation of San Antonio. I happened upon it when I was visiting that city shortly after New Year's, driving around in a daze from sampling the first of some 150 different tortillas that I eventually tasted for this story. Through the door behind the retail counter, I could see women and men in casual clothes and hair nets tending to presses and conveyor belts as corn tortillas streamed by.

"Do you think I could come watch the process?" I asked the clerk. "You'll have to see the boss," he said. A minute later I was shown into the office of the factory's owner, 73-year-old Jesús Villarreal, who was reading the morning paper amid stacks of papers and file boxes. He said he would be delighted to show me around at six the next morning, three hours into the company's daily routine. It makes 630,000 tortillas a week for walk-in retail customers and 94 local restaurants.

In important ways Sanitary is a relic of the past. To begin with, its workers cook the corn on the premises, heating it with lime (calcium oxide) in a process that has been used in Mexico for thousands of years. (Alkali processing causes a chemical reaction that frees up the niacin in the kernels, making the treated grain actually more nutritious than fresh corn.) The cooked corn is also ground at the factory, between two volcanic-rock millstones. The third link with the past is not something the factory does but something it doesn't do: add preservatives and dough conditioners. Its thin, pure-corn tortillas—some of which are turned out by a few superannuated original machines that Villarreal keeps running with old bicycle chains and cobbled-together parts—are no different today than they were when the factory was founded in 1925. Said Villarreal: "I was told by the man who started the company that two of these machines were the first automatic tortilla-makers ever used in the United States." More than just a link with the past, the Sanitary tortilla factory is a living museum.

One hundred and fifty miles to the southeast, in Corpus Christi, is a tortilla operation of an entirely different scale: the 20,000-square-foot plant that belongs to the H-E-B supermarket chain. When I visited in February, it was in the midst of making its weekly quota of 12 million corn and flour tortillas, supplying all of the corporation's 275 stores in Texas and Mexico. The factory runs 24 hours a day, seven days a week, keeping seven production lines and 138 employees busy. Unlike my tour of Sanitary, where the boss showed me around and fed me piping-hot tortillas fresh off the line, at H-E-B's big metal building I was escorted by a cadre of four—plant manager Mike Reischman, two operations experts, and a public relations executive—who explained how everything worked (and fed me hot tortillas fresh off the line). H-E-B doesn't grind the corn itself but starts with Maseca-brand dry corn flour (made by the ubiquitous Mission Foods). It also adds preservatives and conditioners to its dough, though not nearly as much, Reischman says, as some companies do. The product that rolls off its assembly lines is a thoroughly modern tortilla.

The ever-expanding tortilla industry is, or soon will be, at a crossroads. As of today, the old and the new, the large and the small, still coexist in Texas. But times are changing, so don't wait forever to make that trip to your little neighborhood *tortillería*. Not long ago, I came across a news item and couldn't help thinking that it was symbolic of what is happening to the business today: Last year the Guinness keeper of the records certified Mama Ninfa's Original Mexican Restaurant in Houston for its achievement in constructing—what else?—the world's largest taco. The specially made tortilla that swaddled the monster's 1,045 pounds of spicy filling measured 32 inches wide by 16 feet long. Now that's big.

*April 2001*

# SLUSH FUN

PATRICIA SHARPE

Restaurateur Mariano Martinez invented the frozen-margarita machine thirty years ago this month. ¡SALUD!

THIRTY YEARS AGO THIS month—on May 11, 1971, to be exact—Dallas restaurateur Mariano Martinez, Jr., opened the spigot of a converted soft-serve ice cream machine and filled a glass with a history-making pale green slush—the world's first mass-produced frozen margarita. Do not misunderstand: The beverage that emerged from the device was not the first frozen margarita ever; the drink had been around since the blender was introduced in the late thirties. No, this naughty cocktail was much more important. This was the party in a tank that fueled the disco era in Texas, jump-started the national Mexican food craze, and raised the status of tequila from a pariah to a prince among alcoholic beverages. Three decades later the stainless-steel appliance that launched a zillion hangovers sits just inside the front door of Mariano's Mexican Cuisine on Greenville Avenue in North Dallas. It may have all the glamour of an iced-tea dispenser, but this is the machine that created the national drink of Texas. It is hard to imagine today, but in the late fifties, when Martinez was a teenager waiting tables at El Charro, his father's Mexican restaurant in Dallas, tequila was unknown to most people in the United States and considered weird by the rest. Flipping through a scrapbook recently in his home office in the city's affluent Lakewood neighborhood, Martinez remembers those long-ago days: "Customers—they were all Anglos—would show up with a bottle of tequila someone had brought them from Mexico and ask my dad, 'What do we do with this?'" The elder Martinez would whip up a batch of frozen margaritas using a recipe he had gotten from a bartender at a private club in San Antonio in the late thirties. Made with fresh-squeezed lime juice, Cointreau, and a secret ingredient, the drinks were quite a hit. "The next thing you knew," Martinez remembers, "the bottle would be empty and the people would be having a great time."

In 1971, after a ten-year stretch during which he dropped out of high school, played in a rock and roll band, raised considerable hell, and ultimately graduated from Dallas's El Centro College, the 26-year-old Martinez decided to open his own Mexican restaurant. "I went to my father," he says, "and asked him if he would give me his special margarita recipe." His dad agreed. "Papa was a hardheaded person, a private person," Martinez says, "and it touched me that he was willing to share it. It brought tears to my eyes." The restaurant opened in April and, thanks to word of mouth and some well-placed free plugs from the gregarious young owner's friends in the broadcast media, it was immediately packed. On the second night, a customer stopped Martinez and asked, "Do you know how to make frozen margaritas?" "Oh, yes, sir, the best," he answered. "Well," the customer growled, "you'd better talk to your bartender, because these are terrible."

Martinez says he went weak in the knees, envisioning imminent failure and the added humiliation of screwing up his father's recipe. It was easy to see what was wrong, though. The bartender was so swamped with orders that he was just throwing ingredients into the blender without measuring them. And he wasn't happy about having to make such a complicated cocktail. When Martinez tried to talk to the man, he blew up and threatened to walk out: "I'm going back to Steak and Ale," he said, "where the customers only want bourbon and Coke or scotch and water."

The next morning on his way to work, a chastened Martinez stopped at a 7-Eleven to buy chewing gum. While he was waiting in line, he noticed some kids ordering Slurpees. Suddenly, out of nowhere, a notion hit him. "It was like I was channeling the idea," he says. "I thought, 'We could premix the margaritas in a Slurpee machine and all the bartender would have to do is pull the lever.'" As soon as he could get to a phone, he called the Southland Corporation, the Dallas-based owner of 7-Eleven, and asked if he could buy a machine. The company representative was suspicious. "No deal," he said. Martinez kept calling around until someone finally told him about a local man named Frank Adams who had been pestering restaurants with a crazy idea for making frozen daiquiris in a machine.

The two met and decided to pool their knowledge. Adams got hold of a soft-serve ice cream machine and started tinkering. Martinez worked on the margarita recipe. It took some experimentation to adjust for large quantities and the fact that the machine did not use ice but water (which it then froze together with all the other ingredients). A couple of weeks later they lugged the contraption into the bar at Mariano's. Because he had nowhere to hide it, Martinez put the clunky machine out in full view. As it turned out, his customers loved the margaritas that poured out in a slithery frozen stream.

In retrospect Martinez's timing couldn't have been better. In a matter of months the Texas Legislature made it legal for restaurants to sell liquor by the drink in their dining rooms instead of in separate "private clubs," and restaurants all over the state started serving cocktails. The combination of booze and a booming economy started the good times rolling, and they didn't slow down for almost ten years. The upper part of Greenville Avenue, centering on the Old Town shopping center, became *the* singles destination in Dallas, and Mariano's bar was happy-hour central. Pictures on the wall show Willie Nelson, Frank Sinatra, Jr., assorted Dallas Cowboys, and the stars of the television series *Dallas* (scenes for the show were filmed there on five occasions). Southern Methodist University's party-hearty contingent practically moved into the cantina. When Bob Hope performed at SMU in the late seventies, he knew how to win over the audience. "I went over to Mariano's for a margarita," he told the crowd. Everybody cheered and whistled. "I won't say how big it was," he continued, "but the glass had a diving board." The students shrieked with laughter. "And," Hope concluded, "they had to put the salt on with a paint roller."

Patricia
Sharpe

Mariano's *was* margaritaville, and its publicity-savvy owner, who sported a mustache and goatee and was given to appearing at public functions like charity events wearing a Mexican bandido outfit, became quite the local celebrity. The economic and public-relations value of his creation did not go unnoticed either. Other restaurants and clubs quickly copied his idea, and by the end of the seventies, the drink machine was required equipment in any big bar. In 1984 Martinez received a commendation from the Association of Tequila Producers (a now-defunct trade group) for putting tequila on the map in the United States. In 1996, on the twenty-fifth anniversary of the invention of the machine, both the City of Dallas and the Texas House of Representatives passed resolutions of appreciation. Martinez estimates that in the first year, when the concoction was still a novelty, nine out of ten drinks he sold were margaritas.

Martinez never tried to patent his innovation. "I was too busy running the restaurant," he says, "and at the time, it didn't seem like that big a deal." His associate Frank Adams developed a nice little business leasing frozen-drink machines for a while, but once the initial collaboration was over, the two went their separate ways. (The last Martinez heard, Adams was living in Florida.) Late in 1971, after combating continual problems with the margaritas' consistency and discovering that some of his bartenders were selling the recipe behind his back, Martinez had a commercial drink-mix company come up with a formula. That way the recipe would remain secret and there would be no variation from batch to batch. The formula makes concessions to mass production, using high-quality lemon and lime concentrates and corn syrup, common in the soft-drink business because it is cheaper than cane sugar. In the restaurant the bottled liquid is mixed with Cuervo Gold Especial tequila, Cointreau, and his dad's secret ingredient, of course. (The top-shelf or "Texas margarita" also has Grand Marnier.) I tried one of these babies the other day, and I have to say that while it may not be a handcrafted margarita with freshly squeezed Mexican-lime juice, it had a clean, pleasant taste and it went down real smooth.

This month Martinez will celebrate the thirtieth anniversary of his creation with a margaritafest at his six Dallas-area restaurants—three Mariano's and three La Hacienda Ranches. If you order a frozen margarita between May 5 and 11, your first drink will be the same size and price it was in 1971—six ounces for $1.25. It will not, however, emerge from a dinky, 1971-era dispenser. At the huge La Hacienda Ranch in Colleyville, for instance, three flavors (original, strawberry, and Texas) will be dispensed from four ever-churning tanks. The tanks will never run out because they will be continuously refilled by hoses leading from twenty-gallon containers of margarita mix discreetly hidden in a walk-in cooler.

No doubt plenty of people will show up for the event, and no doubt plenty of them will remember the old days, when the customers at Mariano's on Greenville Avenue wore miniskirts and leisure suits, the cocktail waitresses wore hot pants, and—when the mood and the margs were just right—the musicians in the cantina would coax the revelers to their feet and everybody would snake-dance out the front door, disappearing into the margaritaville night.

*May 2001*

# THE SHUCK STOPS HERE

PATRICIA SHARPE

'Tis the season for tamales, but we Texans love them at any time of the year. From their ancient beginnings to mail-order sources to how to make them yourself, here's everything you need to know about these morsels *muy sabrosos.*

WHEN MY FRIEND HORTENCIA "Tense" Vitali was growing up in Laredo in the seventies, tamale making was a Thanksgiving ritual as keenly anticipated as the holiday itself. As I listened to her stories of the fun that she and her siblings had helping her mother prepare mountains of these savory treats, I felt quite deprived that I had not grown up in a large Hispanic family. "There were ten of us kids," says Tense, who is now 38 and an Austin interior designer, "plus a cook, a housekeeper, and of course my mom and dad, and even my littlest brothers and sisters had their part to do. It was a huge affair."

The preparations began two days before T-Day, when Candelaria Cisneros and a contingent of her children would drive downtown to La Fe, "a big, old ceiling fan–cooled masa factory," to pick up her order of the corn dough that would enclose the tamales' central filling. Mrs. Cisneros was particular about quality and insisted on finely ground white masa, not yellow, which she considered inferior. Because this was before the widespread use of dehydrated masa, factories like La Fe started with real corn, and a warm, almost sweet aroma emanated from dozens of dough mixers. The next stop was the butcher shop, where Mrs. Cisneros picked up a whole, cut-up pig—head, feet, and all. The shoulder meat would be set aside for the tamales and the rest frozen for other uses such as barbacoa. Then it was across the border to Nuevo Laredo's open-air market to sift through piles of dried corn husks, strings of garlic, cinnamon sticks, and dark red ancho chiles.

When they got back home, Mrs. Cisneros tied on her apron and began the serious work of cooking the pork and getting the masa ready. The next day the family tamale team was marshaled, with plenty of hot chocolate on hand for the children and beer for the adults. It was a regular assembly line. "We had the ones who soaked the corn husks to make them pliable and pulled off the silk," says Tense, "then the ones who spread the masa on the husks." Another person carefully put a dab of chile-and-cumin-seasoned meat and exactly three raisins in each of the bite-size tamales, and still others rolled and tucked the shucks into the familiar tubular shape. The last one stacked them in the steamers. As many as 55 dozen would be made at Thanksgiving, both the pork version and cinnamony, raisin-filled sweet tamales, and half of them would be frozen for Christmas. There was no such thing as too many tamales. After the interminable hour that it took them to steam on top of the stove, the first ones were gingerly unwrapped and eaten, straight from the shucks.

Tamales are fiesta food. In Hispanic communities throughout the United States, they signal times for celebration, such as New Year's and Mexico's two independence days, el Cinco de Mayo and el Diez y Seis de Septiembre. They are also obligatory for more solemn occasions like el Día de los Muertos (the Day of the Dead) on November 1 and 2, when departed loved ones are remembered with home altars decorated with the honoree's favorite things (a vase of lilies, a Spurs jersey, a bottle of Tecate). But these masa snacks don't require a holiday to be enjoyed; bowls and platters brimming with them also make their appearance at birthdays, wedding showers, and family reunions. In other words, at the kinds of events where Anglos would typically be milling about balancing a plate of finger sandwiches and a glass of wine, chances are tradition-minded Latinos will be peeling the husks off tamales.

Tamales are among the most ancient foods of the New World, dating back at least two thousand years. To the Maya, who lived in and around what is now Central America and Mexico's Yucatán Peninsula, the tamale was the cultural equivalent of our cheese-burger. A graceful drawing on a vase discovered at the ruins of Tikal, in Guatemala, shows a well-fed noble in a feather headdress sitting cross-legged in front of a bowl of neatly rolled tamales. It was the Aztecs of central Mexico, though, who were the masters of the tamale universe, making the handy packages in a multitude of shapes (little canoes, animals) and colors of masa (white, red, yellow). Chile-spiked turkey and dog meat were favorite fillings. The word "tamale"—the correct singular form in Spanish is *tamal*, by the way—is derived from "tamalli," a word in the Aztec language, Nahuatl.

Although many elements of Mexico's indigenous cultures vanished forever with the coming of the conquistadores in 1519, tamales survived. In fact, if it hadn't been for the Spanish and the boatloads of squealing pigs they brought with them, modern-day tamales would lack their second most important ingredient after corn: lard, which gives the masa flavor and flexibility. (Pre-Hispanic tamales were more like thick steamed tortillas—"tender and quivery," in the words of cookbook author Rick Bayless.) To-day the variety of tamales made in Mexico and other parts of the Latin world is astonishing. Around Tampico, in eastern Mexico, giant *sacahuiles*, swathed in banana leaves and big enough for a whole pork loin, emerge from adobe ovens. In Sinaloa, in the western part of the country, tamales of almost equal girth are filled with a veritable stew of pork, zucchini, potatoes, green beans, plantains, and serrano chiles. The far southern state of Chiapas has its iguana tamales. In her cookbook *The Cuisines of Mexico*, Diana Kennedy wrote of tamales from coastal Campeche that are made with a near-transparent dough, "so delicate that it trembles at a touch."

But as vast and intriguing as these varieties may be, we Texans know what a tamale is, and we're not messing with it. It's true that certain modern American chefs, Dallas's own Stephan Pyles among them, have played fast and loose with the whole notion, making masa-less tamales of arborio rice pudding or apples in brioche pastry that would startle even the ancient Aztecs. But for most of us, whatever our heritage, the familiar, homely cylinder of masa remains the gold standard. We may flirt with exotic types, but in these uncertain times there is much to be said for simplicity, for the ritual of opening a corn husk-wrapped bundle and letting its steamy contents tumble onto our plate. We take a bite of that soft masa coating with its filling of moist, chile-spiked pork and pause. Ah, yes. For a moment, at least, all seems right with the world.

### TAMALES 101

Inspired by Tense's childhood memories, I decided to make tamales one night. In the course of doing so, I consulted half a dozen Mexican-food cookbooks and also validated Murphy's Law (everything that could go wrong did). My tamales looked like miniature loofahs (oddly shaped and full of little holes), but they tasted great. Here are some tips that I gleaned from the process, so that you too can make tamales even if you don't have a Mexican grandmother to answer questions.

**Shopping list.** Most ingredients can be found at supermarkets (try the produce section or Mexican-products section for corn husks). Fiesta Mart sells ready-made masa for 50 cents a pound (specify masa for tamales, which is more coarsely ground than tortilla masa). So do tortilla factories and grocery stores in Hispanic neighborhoods. Here is the list of factories.

### AUSTIN

DOS HERMANOS TORTILLA FACTORY AND RESTAURANT, 2730 E. Cesar Chavez (E. First), 512-474-9655. This simple, brightly painted little factory on the east side has a handful of packaged goods like *mole* for sale, as well as pan dulce ("sweet bread") in astonishing colors, and a tiny restaurant on the side. It feels like Mexico in here (ratings: corn 3, flour 4).

EL MILAGRO OF TEXAS TORTILLA FACTORY, 910 E. Sixth, 512-477-
6476. This storefront hops on weekends, when customers line up
to get giant bags of chips for parties, masa dough for tamales, and
baked goods. Mexican polka music blares out a cheery bip-bip-
bip. White corn tortilla rating: 4. Yellow corn: 2.5. Flour: 4 (the
factory makes spinach and tomato as well as plain).

## DALLAS

LUNA'S TORTILLAS, 1615 McKinney Avenue, 214-747-2661. Founded
in 1924 by Maria Luna and run by her grandson Juan Luna, this
factory makes 120,000 corn and flour tortillas daily for hotels,
restaurants, and other corporate clients (ratings: corn 3.5, flour 3).
Anyone can stop by for tortillas, masa, chorizo, pan dulce ("sweet
bread"), and other goodies. Breakfast taquitos in warm flour tortillas cost a mere $1.35 each.

## EL PASO

LA ROTATIVA TORTILLA FACTORY, 2010 Montana Avenue, 915-533-
2317. Because the thin corn tortillas made at this factory have no
preservatives or dough conditioners (chemicals and enzymes that
improve the dough's texture), they have a pure, almost nutty flavor, but they also dry out quickly (rating: 3). Thinner than other
local flour tortillas, La Rotativa's stand out for excellent flavor and
fine layers (4).

TEMO Y TEKA TORTILLA FACTORY, 172 N. Moon Road, Socorro,
915-858-9479. It's hard to imagine better flour tortillas than these
big, thin, golden circles with brown splotches from the grill. They
taste buttery (though it's bound to be lard) and tear easily (rating: 5).
The soft, thinnish corn tortillas are equal to restaurant quality (4).
Mexican food to go too.

VALLE REAL, 11881 Socorro Road, San Elizario, 915-851-0333. This
factory's teensy corn tortillas are real cuties, with a sweet, toasted
flavor (rating: 5). Its oversized flour tortillas are so puffy they're
like dinner rolls (4). But the real specialties are the corn-flour-and-

whole-wheat tortillas, which have a unique texture that makes them seem more like crackers than tortillas (4).

## FORT WORTH

CARDONA FOODS, 850 Meacham Boulevard, 817-625-6477. This longtime commercial tortilla factory in an industrial park northwest of downtown became a hot lunch place a few years ago. The smooth, somewhat thick corn tortillas bear tread marks from the machine belt (rating: 3); the soft flour tortillas are run-of-the-mill (rating: 2.5).

MARQUEZ, 1730 E. Division, Arlington, 817-265-8858. The late Jose Marquez, a poor immigrant from Piedras Negras, built a multimillion-dollar bakery operation in San Angelo, Odessa, and Arlington. Today his family's Arlington factory turns out more than 10,000 flour tortillas daily (rating: 3.5). You can buy them in bulk or enjoy one as a hot, soft-but-sturdy jacket for your breakfast burrito in the bakery's airy little cafe.

RODRIGUEZ FESTIVE FOODS, 899 N. Houston, 817-624-2123. This commercial supplier also sells retail customers average-quality corn and flour tortillas (rating: 3).

## HOUSTON

AYALA'S TORTILLA FACTORY, 5616 Fulton, 713-691-2676. Although Ayala's is just a factory and not much to look at, it does sell retail. Its tender Torti-Mex brand flour tortillas—with a top layer that actually separates to form a pocket, like pita bread—are far better than the typical mass-produced version (rating: 4). Its corn tortillas are pretty average (2.5).

LA POBLANA TORTILLA FACTORY, 7648 Canal, 713-921-4760. If you don't eat more of these tender, golden flour tortillas than you intended, you just aren't hungry (rating: 4.5). The lovely, soft corn tortillas are addictive (4.5). Allow time to grab a taco or a plate of good carnitas (pork tips) at the appealing, ultracasual restaurant up front.

SANDY'S FLOUR TORTILLAS, 5711 McPherson, 956-727-7441. The entrance to this strip-mall spot is inconspicuous, but the factory inside is huge and bustling. Basic flour tortillas (rating: 3) are sold raw, to be cooked at home. Local restaurants El Taco Tote and Danny's buy custom-made tortillas from Sandy's.

## RIO GRANDE VALLEY

DON PEDRO'S, 4120 N. Twenty-third, McAllen, 956-686-8936. In the small restaurant in front of the factory, everything from fragrant pan dulce (sweet bread) to barbacoa is sold. Even though the space is basic, carved Mexican furniture perks it up. The corn tortillas are average (rating: 3), but the thin, multilayered flour tortillas rise above the norm (4).

EMILIA'S RESTAURANT, 605 W. Elizabeth, 956-504-9899; and 5182 E. Fourteenth, 965-838-2221, Brownsville. The heavenly smell of corn envelops you when you walk into the tortilla factories at the back of these two bright, cheery restaurants. One of the monster flour tortillas will fill you up (rating: 4), but you'll need more of the teensy and oddly salty corn ones (3).

EXQUISITA TORTILLAS, 700 W. Chapin, Edinburg, 956-383-3011. Valley residents are big fans of Exquisita, a local brand sold in grocery stores. The factory is on Chapin Street, but you can also get the products, plus tacos and pan dulce ("sweet bread"), at the company's Tacofé restaurant-bakeries in McAllen (525 N. Twenty-third and 703 Dove) and Edinburg (320 N. Twelfth). The medium-thin corn tortillas are good (rating: 3), the nicely layered flour versions better (4).

GARZA'S TORTILLA FACTORY, 1010 S. F, Harlingen, 956-425-3313. The affiliated restaurant next door has a big local following for its barbacoa, even though it is near a highway and very basic. The corn tortillas are standard but good (rating: 3). Garza's does not make flour tortillas, but other companies' brands are sold here.

Patricia
Sharpe

LIMON'S TORTILLERIA, 34 U.S. 281, 956-544-2969; and 603 E. Jefferson, 956-542-8497, Brownsville. Tiny and painted yellow, Limon's factory could pass for a Mexican raspa (snow cone) stand. Most people use the drive-through; you can smell the corn from your car. Locals like these mild, standard-quality tortillas for making nachos and migas (rating: 3).

TREVIÑO'S RESTAURANT AND TORTILLA FACTORY, 54 Boca Chica Boulevard, Brownsville, 956-544-7866. Treviño's is a bit out of the way (you'll pass the intersection called the triangle if you're coming from downtown; look for a former convenience store with old gas pumps outside), but you can get excellent, almost pita-like flour tortillas here (rating: 4.5) and grab a taco in the unprepossessing restaurant.

SAN ANTONIO

ADELITA TAMALES AND TORTILLA FACTORY, 1130 Fresno, 210-733-5352. In a tidy, painted cinder-block building near I-10, you'll find this little tortilla factory with a neighborhood clientele. Its flour tortillas, with a good, fresh taste (rating: 4), are better than the slightly stiff corn (3). Adelita also sells masa, barbacoa, and bundles of steaming tamales.

SANITARY TORTILLA MANUFACTURING CORPORATION, 623 Urban Loop, near I-35; 210-226-9209. Although both corn and flour tortillas are sold, only the corn are made at this simple place, one of the oldest factories in the city. Quite thin, with good corn flavor, they are also admirably pure, having no preservatives or additives (rating: 3.5). Tamales, masa, chicharrones, and other foods are sold to go.

**Wrap stars.** You can use a variety of waterproof wrappers to hold the tamale while it cooks: corn shucks, banana leaves, avocado leaves, even plastic wrap. (The latter is a little soulless, but it works great for those odd shapes; you peel it off before serving.) Corn shucks are the most common in Texas, though, so I'll concentrate on them. To make dried shucks pliable, soak them in a

bowl of very hot water for thirty minutes, weighting them with a
saucer so they don't float. (For a pretty holiday presentation, soak
them in red hibiscus tea.) Fresh shucks can be used too.

**Critical masa.** I tried making a few tamales with the fresh
ready-made masa that I bought at Fiesta. But I was much hap-
pier with the less dense masa I whipped up myself using dry masa
harina (again, be sure to get the kind that is specifically for tamales). It was light, almost spongy, and the whole process was as easy
as using a cake mix. Maseca is a good brand, but the package instructions aren't very detailed. So here are some wise words from
the experts:

For meat-filled tamales, mix your masa harina with lard and
warm chicken stock, using amounts specified on the package; for
sweet tamales, use vegetable shortening and warm water. Which-
ever fat you use, chill it for an hour or so and beat it with a mixer
for at least a minute to make it light and fluffy. After you mix the
dry masa with warm liquid, add it in batches to the beaten fat.
Continue beating the dough for one to three minutes until it is
approximately the texture of a butter-cream frosting. The dough
is ready if a teaspoon-size chunk floats in a cup of cold water. (A
word about lard. I know what you're thinking: "Yech! Pig fat. No
way." But it's lower in cholesterol and saturated fat than butter
and lower in trans-fats than shortening. It's also clean and pure
white—and meat-filled tamales just don't taste right without it.)

**General assembly.** Every cookbook has a different masa-
spreading method: Spread it on the middle of the corn husk; no,
spread it on the lower half. Cover the husk all the way to the sides;
no, leave margins. The truth is, they all work. Here's the best way I
found to make the typical cylindrical Tex-Mex tamale. Pat a corn
husk dry and lay it in front of you (if some are too small, overlap
two of them and use a dab of masa to stick them together). With
a knife or a spatula, spread a scant one-fourth cup of masa into a
four-inch square (these measurements do not need to be exact).
Leave a border of about two inches at the pointy end of the husk
and three fourths of an inch on the other three sides. Spoon your
filling of choice down the middle of the square, then lift the two
sides of the husk, bring them together to encase the filling, and

fold them both to the left. Then fold the pointy flap over them like the flap on an envelope. The other end stays open, but if you prefer, you can fold it over too; just leave more of a margin at that end when you're smearing on the dough. The finished tamales look cute when tied with thin strips of husk or colored ribbon, but this isn't necessary.

By the way, there's nothing sacred about the usual stogie form. You can make tamales any size or shape your heart desires—circular, square, triangular, crescent-shaped, whatever. Mention this when your friends convulse with laughter over your efforts.

**Now you're cooking.** Steaming is the most common way of cooking tamales, in a tamale cooker, a vegetable steamer, or whatever you can improvise. Stack the tamales upright in the top part of the steamer, open ends up. Spread extra husks between each layer. Pack the tamales firmly but not tightly, and put a wet, wrung-out dishtowel on the top layer to absorb water that condenses on the lid. Cover the pan and steam for 45 minutes to 2 hours; the time varies tremendously depending on how many you're cooking and how big they are. Several cookbook authors suggest putting a penny in the water when you start heating it; if it stops dancing about, add more boiling water *fast*. If the steam is interrupted before your tamales are cooked, they will fall like a cake and be heavy. The tamales are done when the husks come away cleanly from the dough. Let them rest for 5 to 10 minutes in the steamer before serving. To reheat tamales, either leave them in their husks and resteam for 2 to 5 minutes, depending on the quantity; wrap them in foil and put them in a 350-degree oven or toaster oven (allow about 20 minutes for half a dozen); or heat them individually in their husks on an ungreased comal or skillet over a low flame. Microwaving tends to make them tough.

**By the book.** Here are my favorite cookbooks for tamales, and they're fun to read too: *Rick Bayless's Mexican Kitchen: Capturing the Vibrant Flavors of a World-Class Cuisine* (Scribner, 1996, hardcover, 448pp.); Diana Kennedy's *The Essential Cuisines of Mexico: Revised and updated throughout, with more than 30 new recipes* (Clarkson Potter, 2000, hardcover, 544 pp.); Mark Miller, Stephan Pyles, and John Sedlar's *Tamales!* (Wiley, 1st edition,

2003, paperback, 192pp.); and Zarela Martínez's *Food From My Heart: Cuisines of Mexico Remembered and Reimagined* (Wiley, 1995, paperback, 346 pp.).

*November 2001*

# HOW SWEET IT IS

SUZY BANKS

Ve said they were cool. Would you believe cold? But even a late freeze can't dampen our enthusiasm for peaches, the juiciest crop of the summer.

BLUEFFORD HANCOCK SQUEEZED MY ELBOW as if testing it for ripeness—an understandable gesture, considering that he was in the midst of appraising peaches at the fortieth annual Stonewall Peach JAMboree, where he has served as a judge since the festival's inception. A retired horticulturist with the Texas Cooperative Extension, a branch of Texas A&M University, Hancock remained focused on the task at hand, refusing to be distracted by my elbow, the late-June heat, or even the dance recital on a nearby stage, where waist-high cuties decked out in indigo sequins hammed it up to "Has Anybody Seen My Gal?" He bestowed blue ribbons on the cream of the crop, like the heaviest peach (a .79-pound Harvester, rather wimpy compared with past winners that weighed in at more than a pound) and the prettiest one (another Harvester).

But Hancock, who helped start the Texas Peach Growers Association in 1952, knows that the real measure of a winning peach is more than skin-deep. "It's about how they taste, and Texas peaches taste the best," he said, unable to resist a dig at that nefarious farming state out west, whose peaches "look like a magazine cover photo and taste like wallpaper paste."

A little gloating can be forgiven, since this scene took place two years ago, when Texas peaches were plentiful. Then last year a late freeze reduced the crop to a third of the average 30 million pounds, and this summer's harvest will be even smaller, thanks to a particularly devastating freeze at the end of March.

Amid such a paucity of peaches, it's hard to imagine that there was a time when the peaches-for-fun-and-profit craze consumed East Texas landowners much like tulipomania infected seventeenth-century Holland. It all began sanely enough around 1890, when the state's first commercial crop rolled out of the area surrounding Tyler, which boasted ideal growing conditions as well as rail lines leading to northern markets. At the turn of the century, the area's cotton farmers were hit with the double whammy of falling prices and a boll weevil invasion. Meanwhile, wildly exaggerated reports of the easy money to be made growing peaches spurred thousands of farmers—not to mention lawyers, merchants, and doctors—to sink everything into peach orchards. Although 90 percent of the would-be orchardists had no fruit-growing experience, the sheer number of trees they planted, coupled with the absence of modern-day diseases and pests, made up for their agricultural ignorance, and in 1912 East Texas was buried under 149.9 million pounds of the fruit. The surplus of peaches— mainly Elbertas—was so large that there weren't enough railcars to haul them north, and millions of pounds were piled along the railroad right-of-way to rot. But like some mutation from a fifties horror flick, the peaches couldn't be stopped: The bumper crop of 1919 topped 221 million pounds.

Eventually, mountains of rotting peaches and prices of pennies per bushel not only thinned the herd of pomologists but also motivated true believers to find solutions to this wasteful bounty. Horticulturists researched varieties that would ripen in sequence throughout a longer season, and now we have cling peaches like Springold and Regal that ripen in mid-May, semi-freestones like Juneprince and Gala that take over in early June, and the beloved freestones, such as Harvester, Loring, Dixiland, and Parade, that carry us halfway through August.

Gradually, peach trees crept west across Texas, taking root mainly in a wide central swath from Dallas to the Hill Country.

Parker County, west of Fort Worth, claims the title Peach Capital of Texas, and De Leon, in nearby Comanche County, is home to the long-running Peach and Melon Festival, now in its eighty-ninth year. Growers in the Valley have even tried their hand at the crop but with limited success. David Byrne, however, a professor of horticulture at Texas A&M who has developed several varieties that are compatible with mild winters, holds high hopes for the region.

While the Tyler area still produces its share of the blushing fruit, it has dropped to number two in the state in production. The leader is now the renowned Gillespie County, which has the kind of dirt (red-clay subsoil topped with potassium-rich sandy loam) that peaches love, according to Bluefford Hancock. While crowing about the caliber of their crop seems to be required of peach farmers throughout the universe, nowhere is the chest-thumping louder than in this Hill Country county.

Don't go to the Gold Orchards farm stand, on U.S. 290, for instance, and ask for Fredericksburg peaches. You're in Stonewall, locally considered the birthplace of Hill Country peach farming. As far as the Golds and most other Stonewall growers are concerned, those gentlemen farmers over in Fredericksburg, fifteen miles west, merely dabble in the business.

The Golds weren't the first farming family in Gillespie County to plow under their peanuts and plant peaches commercially. (That distinction goes to B. L. Enderle, who reportedly kick-started the local industry back in the mid-twenties.) But the family has been at it steadily for three generations now. The late Erwin Gold planted a few peach trees on his land just northwest of Stonewall proper in 1940 and sold his harvest on the roadside from the trunk of his 1937 Ford sedan. By the early seventies, Erwin—with help from his wife, Alma, and their three strapping sons, Alvin, Harley, and Lawrence—was picking 20,000 bushels of peaches in good years and tending to more than two hundred acres of the handsome little trees.

Harley, 73, and Lawrence, 63, claim to be retired (Alvin passed away in 1999), having handed the reins to Lawrence's daughter, Luana Priess, and her husband, Ricky. But the brothers can't stay away from the family's farm stand for long. That's where I caught up with them back in 2001, just as a trailerload of Lorings arrived to begin their journey through the forty-foot-long grading machine, a contraption that marries the beauty of automation with human judgment.

As the peaches jostled down the grader's first conveyor belt, the overripe and severely blemished were culled by hand. Those that made the cut were then defuzzed with water and spinning brushes. Next, the buffed beauties danced along a section of rotating sponges that gently dried them before another conveyor belt carried them through a second gauntlet of inspection. Like proud parents, Lawrence and Ricky searched for the slightest imperfections; just a dab of infectious brown rot on one peach can spread through a bushel of the fruit faster than gossip in a small town. Finally, the survivors—the Gold standard, if you will—were sorted by size in an ingenious device that reminded me of a carnival game, with a grinning Harley checking the fruit one last time for nearly microscopic defects. Throughout the entire process, the three men appeared on the verge of giggling.

I have to confess that, until I saw the magical grading machine, I didn't understand how peach farming could appeal to anyone but a die-hard masochist, even in the best of times. Sure, as I toured the Golds' lush orchards, with their trees lined up precisely, like a vast, bright-green army, I thought how cool it would be to coax bounty from the earth and all that. But any romantic notions I had died when the talk turned to root rot and other diseases, creepy insects like stinkbugs, drought, floods, hailstorms, too few chilling hours (between 32 and 45 degrees) to set the fruit and too few sunny days to sweeten it—not to mention those cruel late freezes.

And that's not all: You have to wait four years after planting the trees to harvest your first crop. The real kicker, though, was learning that, in those rare years when everything comes together perfectly and the trees are heavily burdened with fruit, about a fourth of the baby peaches must be plucked or shaken off for the sake of the others. Murder! And if you think I'm neurotically tenderhearted, even Jim Kamas, a fruit specialist with the Texas Cooperative Extension, likens the task to "stepping on chicks."

The Golds' work doesn't stop in the orchard or at the grading machine. Lynette, Lawrence's wife, sets a breakneck pace in the farm stand's kitchen, which, on the day I visited, was as spotless as one in a model home even though she and her two helpers were busily canning preserves, feeding homemade peach ice cream into the soft-serve machine, and baking a couple dozen pies. Luana was also in the kitchen that day, but she didn't look comfortable in this dauntingly domestic scene. "There's no place she'd rather be than out in the orchard with her father, driving the tractor or whatever," Lynette explained. "She's the son we never had." This make-believe son, however, was gal enough to be a duchess in the JAMboree Peach Court of 1985. Just don't ask her to taste the cash crop. "I love to work with peaches," Luana confessed, "but I hate to eat them."

And they say irony is dead, I thought, as I polished off my second piece of pie. This family sideline—Lynette's brainchild, born four years ago—has taken off faster than you can say "flaky cinnamon crust." During the JAMboree, they sell more than sixty pies a day. Luckily, Lynette, a petite woman with the energy of a hummingbird and the rainy-day instincts of the proverbial ant, is prepared for this year's crop flop. When I checked in with her in April, she assured me that if, as expected, Gillespie County peaches are scarcer than minimalist B&B's this summer, there will still be pies aplenty. Her five big freezers are packed with more than a thousand gallons of bagged and labeled peaches that she has stockpiled in better years. She even has enough to sell to the Stonewall Chamber of Commerce so they'll have something to serve with the ice cream at this year's JAMboree (June 20 and 21).

But even at the 2001 JAMboree, the peach pickings were shockingly slim: store-bought ice cream topped with frozen peaches, doughy cobbler, peach freezes with more vanilla than fruit. No shortage of nachos and sausage-on-a-stick, though (maybe Luana was in charge of the food). I envied the pie-and-cobbler judges, who were happily sampling dozens of entries, safely cordoned off from peach-deprived fairgoers like me.

Cleansing their palates with soda crackers between bites, the lucky judges rated the contenders on appearance, peachiness, and crust. Betty Nebgen, who was standing nearby—she was in charge

*Suzy Banks* of the contest for 21 years before passing the mantle to Marjorie Otte in 2000—explained the rules to me: No pie or cobbler can include ingredients that require refrigeration, like cream cheese, and entries are disqualified if the taste of peaches is overwhelmed by, say, too many almonds or, in the case of one entry a few years ago, Red Hots. "The Red Hots gave the pie a real pretty color," said a diplomatic Nebgen, "and it tasted real good. But not like peaches."

Maybe I could get my piece of the pie at the festival's peach auction, I thought, where the top winners in all the categories— from fresh peaches to jams and jellies—are sold to the highest bidder (a portion of the proceeds goes to the chamber of commerce). But when I watched the heaviest peach go for a whopping $500 and the prettiest one for a princely $600, I realized that my chances of snagging even the fifth-place cobbler were hopeless. I wonder, though, if I'd known then what I know now—that Texas peaches are fragile treasures that we should never take for granted—would any price have seemed too high?

*June 2003*

# TEX-MEX IOI

PATRICIA SHARPE

Nachos, tomatillo sauce, *chile con queso*—will the real Mexican food please stand up? A crash course in Texans' favorite fusion fare.

I'M WRITING THIS COLUMN to apologize for having laughed at my friend and colleague Sam Gwynne. (I was laughing *with* you, Sam. Honest.) A recovering Yankee, Sam has made enormous progress in understanding the behavior and tribal customs of Texans during the nine years he's lived here. But there is one thing he just can't seem to get a handle on: As he put it recently, "What the hell is the difference between Mexican food and Tex-Mex?" Sam has been tragically misinformed that all sorts of popular dishes are Tex-Mex—quesadillas, breakfast tacos, charro beans, black beans, tomatillo sauce, flan, and sopaipillas, to name a few. His questions always make my day, but the afternoon he appeared at my office door to ask plaintively, "Are jalapeños Tex-Mex?" I knew he needed serious help. So, for Sam and everybody else who didn't have the good fortune to get here before 1970, here's my short course on the cuisine that was fusion before fusion was hip.

*Austin, circa 1955:* I'm with my two best friends from junior high school, Laura Ellen and Mary Jean. As they regularly do, Laura Ellen's parents, Mr. and Mrs. Glass, have taken us out to eat Mexican food at El Toro (where the Clay Pit restaurant is now), a big, bustling space filled with tables and vinyl booths and with a large bullfight painting on one wall. While scanning the

Patricia
Sharpe

menu (which we have all but memorized), we pass the time eating saltines, supplied in cellophane wrappers, and hot corn tortillas, which we butter, salt, and roll up like cigars. There are no chips. Mr. Glass spoons a little of the thin, tomatoey hot sauce onto his crackers. Like the waiters, the restaurant's owner, Monroe Lopez, is of Mexican descent. Most of the customers wolfing down rolled-up tortillas are Anglo. The dining room could be the supporting cast for *The Adventures of Ozzie and Harriet*.

Mr. and Mrs. Glass each get a beer (margaritas had not made the scene yet). Then they order combination plates: yellow-cheese-and-onion enchiladas, pork tamales, an ocean of ground-beef *chile con carne* (seasoned with red chile, garlic, and lots of cumin), re-fried beans, and Spanish rice. Laura Ellen has crispy tacos filled with hamburger meat (seasoned with garlic and a little chile) and topped with rapidly warming lettuce and chopped tomato. Mary Jean gets puffy tacos filled with the same thing. (Definitions are in order here: A crispy taco was—is—made with a hard-fried, folded-over corn tortilla; a puffy taco is a corn tortilla that has been fried so that its layers delicately separate and balloon out.) I get *chalupas compuestas*, two crisp-fried flat corn tortillas topped with refried beans, melted yellow cheese, lettuce, and tomato. My friends and I are so filled with anticipation we can hardly sit still.

Our harried waiter warns, "Hotplatehotplate!"—spoken as a single word—as he slides the platters onto the table and checks to see that our tortilla basket is full. Twenty minutes of contented munching ensues. At the end of the meal, he reappears to leave the check and inquire, "Sherbetorcandy?" Did we want a dish of sherbet (pineapple, lime, or orange) or a crisp (not chewy) pecan praline for dessert? That was pretty much what we ate every time. There were no chicken enchiladas in *chipotle* sauce, no flautas with guacamole and sour cream, no *tacos al carbón*. None of the dishes that are now so common would become mainstream in Mexican restaurants here for at least another fifteen years. But in case you're feeling sorry for us, don't. At home, we were all eating tuna casserole, lime Jell-O, and frozen TV dinners. We would have sooner skipped church than our weekly Mexican food fix.

What I like to call classic Tex-Mex was born in Texas in the Mexican restaurants run by first- and second-generation immigrants during the first third of the twentieth century. It peaked in a kind of golden age (the color of melted Velveeta, no doubt) that lasted roughly from World War II to the Vietnam War. During this two- to three-decade span, the spicy components of the combination plate became our most treasured, and most Texan, comfort food. Going out for enchiladas and tacos was a cultural ritual that bound us together as surely as gathering for turkey, dressing, and pumpkin pie at Thanksgiving. By the seventies, though, the winds of change were blowing, and as streams of new Mexican immigrants moved north, bringing with them their more varied and, yes, more exciting interior styles of cooking, classic Tex-Mex began a slow, inexorable fade into the background.

What put the Tex in Tex-Mex? Three things: American yellow cheese, *chile con carne*, and the infinite malleability of the corn tortilla. (Rice and refried beans, while essential, were basically the same rice and beans served in Mexico.) First and foremost, though, is cheese. In Texas during the heyday of Tex-Mex, if it wasn't yellow, it wasn't cheese. Oh, all right—if you looked hard, you could find a few other cheeses, but they lagged far behind yellow cheese in popularity. Knowing what their customers liked, and being no fools, Mexican restaurateurs went with the flow. Most of them used mild American cheese for filling and topping enchiladas; some preferred real cheddar. (Kraft's Velveeta, being utterly bland and easy to melt, was ideal for creating the thin, seasoned sauce called *chile con queso*. So beloved was queso that it took on a life of its own as the national party dip of Texas.) Maybe one in a hundred restaurants used Monterey jack. But even if there had been more-expensive imported Mexican cheeses around, few would have bought them because part of the appeal of Mexican food was that it was cheap. It would have been economic suicide to buck the trend.

The second major component of Tex-Mex is *chile con carne*, a.k.a. chili. The familiar spicy ground-beef stew that we all know and love, or at least tolerate, chili was already a staple in Texas well before the Great Depression of the thirties, when a poor person could buy a filling bowl of it with crackers for a nickel or a dime. Since many Mexican restaurants initially served American dishes too, chili was often already on the menu. Ladling some on

Patricia
Sharpe

a plate of enchiladas wasn't even a stretch, and enchiladas and tamales sauced with *chile con carne* had practically become a basic
food group by the fifties. Some restaurant owners objected that
the combination wasn't "Mexican," and they were right. It was
Texan.

Ah, the tortilla—master of, well, a dozen disguises. Tortillas
go back at least to the Maya and the Aztecs, but it took the cagey
Mexican-food entrepreneurs of the twentieth century and their
deep-fat fryers to fully exploit the tortilla's possibilities. The crispy
taco and the now charmingly archaic puffy taco both emerged
from this felicitous union, but the two most important, and most
Texan, variations on the tortilla were the tortilla chip and, in turn,
its apotheosis, the nacho. It is a fact that until recently, restaurants
in Mexico did not serve either tostadas or nachos as appetizers,
nor did the earliest Mexican restaurants in Texas. These snacks
didn't materialize until sometime around World War II. If you
know a grad student who needs a dissertation topic, tell her or
him to figure out which of the several cafes along the border that
claim to have invented the nacho was actually the first to do it.
That would be a worthy contribution to human knowledge.

One quick final aside. I haven't forgotten the state's most ubiquitous Tex-Mex dish: fajitas. It's quite true that the fajita plate,
with its dramatic sizzle and forest of condiments, was cooked up
in Texas. But fajitas did not become outrageously popular until
1973—when Ninfa's opened in Houston and began selling *tacos al
carbón*—and that was after the classic Tex-Mex era.

Up until thirty years ago, Tex-Mex was the big enchilada at
every Mexican restaurant in the state (sorry, couldn't resist). Our
universe back then was so Tex-centric that people would return
from their first trip to Monterrey or Saltillo griping that they
couldn't get any Mexican food there. It wasn't until travel and the
arrival of new immigrants broadened our worldview that we realized that what we had here wasn't interior Mexican food but a
distinctive regional cuisine that deserved its own name. Luckily,
one was easily appropriated—the catchy term already in use for
the border patois that today we call Spanglish. Today Tex-Mex
has been downsized to a puffy taco, but most Mexican restaurants
serve at least a few dishes. (Some of the most venerable purvey-

ors are Dallas's El Fenix, founded in 1918; Fort Worth's Joe T.
Garcia's, 1935; San Antonio's Mi Tierra, 1941; Houston's Molina's,
1941; and Austin's El Rancho, 1952.) Just scan the menu for words
like "Combinaciones Mexicanas" or "Classic Texas Enchiladas." If
you're of a certain age, order a Señorita Special for old times' sake.
If you're a newcomer, have one out of curiosity. You'll be eating a
part of Texas history.

And, Sam, jalapeños are Tex-Mex only if they're stuffed with
Velveeta.

*August 2003*

# TABLE TALK

## PATRICIA SHARPE

T ex-Mex gets defined by the restaurateurs who made it famous.

## DAVID CORTEZ, MI TIERRA, SAN ANTONIO

I grew up in the business. My father opened the restaurant in 1941;
it was called Jamaica then. I started working there when I was ten
years old. My father came from Guadalajara, and he had an aunt
from there. She was a good cook, and she helped him. She would
tell him what to do.

I would say people started using the term Tex-Mex in the late
sixties, when we started getting a lot of tourists in the city. Tex-
Mex is crisp tacos, cheddar cheese, and puffy tacos. If you eat tamales with cheddar cheese on top, it is more Tex-Mex. If you eat
them with a tomato salsa, it is more Mexican. If you grill them,
that is even more Mexican.

In the old days we did not serve chips on the table. That was
part of the Tex-Mex ambience, and we had to adjust. People would
come in and ask for it. When a lot of people ask for something,
you try to accommodate them. We held out as long as we could,
until the late seventies.

Patricia
Sharpe HOPE GARCIA LANCARTE, JOE T. GARCIA'S,
FORT WORTH

The recipes that we use here came from our mother, Jessie Garcia. She was born in Yurecuaro, Michoacán, in 1905. Her family came to Fort Worth. My father was Joe T. He was born in La Piedad, Michoacán, but my parents didn't meet until they were both in the U.S.

My parents opened the restaurant around 1935. There wasn't that much on the menu in the early days, just barbecue and a Mexican family-style dinner. Joe's barbecue wasn't smoked; it was cooked over charcoal in a pit, which is still there.

A lot of restaurants would put chili over everything, but we did not do that. We still don't. That is not Mexican food. I would say that is Tex-Mex.

I am not insulted by the term Tex-Mex, but I don't like it. That is like chili out of a can. Our chiles rellenos and flautas are like we make them in Mexico.


MATT MARTINEZ, JR., MATT'S EL RANCHO, AUSTIN

We were the only ones who drained our taco meat after we cooked it. A lot of the heartburn from Mexican food is from the fat. Our customers tell us they don't get heartburn from our food. We use a little fat for flavor.

Hot sauce was made famous here. The basic enchilada, taco, rice, beans, and chile relleno—we put it on the map. Back in the old days the big-sell item was tostadas compuestas with guacamole. Tex-Mex is the fastest growing ethnic food in the world.


RAUL MOLINA, JR., FORMER OWNER OF MOLINA'S,
HOUSTON

My dad was from Laredo and so was Mr. Santos Gonzalez—he was the chef. He was with my dad for more than fifty years.

We made our own tortillas in the early days. We had a little machine. At that time, this is going back to the forties during the war, tortilla factories were hard to come by. We found a tortilla company in San Antonio, and we would have tortillas shipped in every morning. That was until Panchos Tortillas opened up in the fifties or early sixties; then they started supplying them to us.

Actually, we made our own kind of chile con queso. Different things evolved—for instance, nachos. I had a bright idea to make the nacho with a round chip, and we asked Pancho's to make them round for us. The nachos were known as the tortilla chip with melted cheese and jalapeños. We added the beans, taco meat, and sour cream—oh boy, dress it up and sell another item. It is all about taking care of your customers.

Most of the recipes were for dishes like the chile gravy, the chile con carne, which was very popular, and the taco meat, the chile con queso, and the Spanish sauce. To this day we still use all of them. At home we ate differently. We ate carne guisada, caldos, and sopas, which we didn't serve at the restaurant.

*August 2003,* Texas Monthly *website*

# GOING FOR THE JIGGLER

ANNE DINGUS

**W**hen I was growing up in the Panhandle, Jell-O played a part in my family's life, and it still does. It's fun, versatile, and always topped with a comforting dollop of nostalgia.

THE RAINBOW TABLE WAS always the best part of the Dingus family reunion. In the big park at little Buffalo Gap, where the clan gathered annually in the fifties and sixties, there were plenty of entertainments for my siblings and me: a swimming pool in which to rinse off the sweat and dirt, older cousins who would take you doodlebug-hunting and rattlesnake-baiting, and a passel of funny names that we snorted about in secret (Aunt Shorty, Uncle Hurschel, Ina Bob). Still, I was most fascinated by the picnic table that bore what seemed like more Jell-O concoctions than there were living Dinguses: dozens of glimmering Pyrex panfuls, their contents melting slightly under the summer sun. Orange, green, yellow, red; coolly translucent or creamily opaque; plain or fruit-choked. Compared with the rest of the food—brown chili, brown beans, brown brownies—they shone in the light like stained-glass windows and, in the children of that era, inspired almost as much reverence, because back then, a portion of Jell-O fit the popular definition of "salad."

Not until the dawn of the seventies did my generation begin to face reality: A true salad involved fresh produce, preferably of the green persuasion. "Jell-O salad," we realized, was, like "mild hot sauce," a Texymoron. This bit of enlightenment—along with more significant cultural shifts, such as the growing demand for organic food—had a chilling effect on our opinion of Jell-O. In response, Jell-O's parent company rethought the food's image as a make-ahead dinner salad and ladies' luncheon specialty. Today, thirty years later, the gelatin giant defines itself as a fun food, more of a child's snack or a low-calorie indulgence. Funny thing, though—when a loved one dies, we still expect friends to drop by with Jell-O offerings, same as always. We're nostalgic about it because we grew up with it. Explaining the enduring appeal of something so venerable, so meaningful, and so multipurpose can be as challenging as, well, nailing Jell-O to a tree.

With the possible exception of the casserole, the Jell-O salad was the ne plus ultra of postwar cuisine. The homecoming of our GIs meant the return of their tool-wielding wives and sweethearts to full feminine status, and many women zestfully reapplied themselves to cooking, cleaning, and home decorating. Jell-O's popularity soared, and it expanded its advertising into television, notably as a sponsor of *I Love Lucy*. My mother, who as a comely twenty-year-old married my ex-Army captain father in 1947, was one of the millions of her generation to become a professional homemaker. Her preferred Jell-O salad involved bing cherries and pecans in black-cherry Jell-O. She centered the square on a lettuce leaf—you didn't have to eat *that*—with a blob of mayonnaise on top (never Miracle Whip; we set the bar high on Mary Ellen Street). This recipe is sometimes called Coke salad because the soft drink can be subbed for the water, but my family would never have squandered a perfectly good Coca-Cola that way.

Those of you with limited exposure to Jell-O cookery may be curling your collective lip right about now, but Mother's salad is, I assure you, a straightforward concept compared with some of the omnium-gelatum recipes I have been served in my day. I'm not talking about the standbys like Golden Glow, lemon Jell-O enhanced with pieces of carrot and pineapple, and Hawaiian Delight, a pick-your-flavor base studded with maraschino cherries, canned pineapple chunks, sliced bananas, miniature marshmallows, slivered almonds, shredded coconut, mango cubes, and tiny leis. (Just kidding. There weren't any mango cubes.) Even more jaw-dropping were such creations as a salad combining lime gelatin, tomato juice, cream cheese, onions, and plums. I've even heard tell of—brace yourself—barbecue Jell-O. Swear to God. It's made with a package of lemon flavor as well as tomato sauce, vinegar, horseradish, salt, and pepper; you chill it, mince it, and sprinkle the bits over salad (the leafy green kind) to accompany brisket or ribs. But I present the Chill-O Award to a dish my friend Lorne Loganbill found in *Feeder's Digest*, a 1977 cookbook from the little town of Canadian. A version of Hawaiian Delight, it's topped with a cooked frosting of sugar, flour, egg, butter, pineapple juice, and whipping cream. Aloha!

Processed gelatin has been around since the early nineteenth century, but back then it was unflavored and came in sheets. One hapless fellow marketed a flavored powder in 1845, but it failed miserably. In 1897 a man named Pearle Wait, of LeRoy, New York, had better luck. His fruit-flavored gelatin tasted good and didn't require chilling, though the thickening took awhile (the concoction was christened "Jell-O" by his wife, whose name was, appropriately, May Wait). Lacking capital, he sold the rights, which eventually ended up the property of a local company, Genesee Pure Foods. Large-scale production began in 1900, and the four flavors—strawberry, raspberry, orange, and lemon—sold for 10 cents a package. Two years later the company racked up a quarter-million dollars in sales.

Timing is everything, of course; ask anyone who's tried to get three supper dishes ready at the same time. Housewives and chefs embraced the new product in part because of its convenience. But a major reason for Genesee's success was its commitment to advertising. The company invested heavily in large print ads—created by such now-renowned illustrators as Norman Rockwell and Maxfield Parrish—that emphasized the simplicity of preparation and featured smiling mothers and children (notably the Jell-O Girl, a winsome blonde with a Dutch bob). Jell-O's bigwigs (bigwiggles?) also boosted sales by associating Jell-O with wealth. In the nineteenth century, gelatin had been the purview of the rich because rendering it from calves' hooves was a complicated procedure requiring several servants. The company milked this upper-class connection in ads that showed elegant females serving Jell-O in champagne flutes at tables set with silver, linens, and tapers.

Gelatin-based fare—all of which quickly came to be known as Jell-O—was considered a classy comestible well into the seventies, and it was a staple of regional cookbooks. A 1949 tome notes that gelatin is "peculiarly appropriate to Texas, coming as it does from cows." Even New York–born Helen Corbitt, the longtime doyenne of Neiman Marcus's famed Zodiac Room, in Dallas, approved of Jell-O, especially as a tonic for the Texas heat and an outlet for housebound wives' creativity. "There is nothing quite as cool as a shimmering molded salad," she wrote in one of her cookbooks, promising amateur chefs that "you may turn out some works of art as your imagination runs riot." And sure enough, the domestic engineers of the era found in "gel cookery"—as one of Jell-O's beleaguered rivals put it—the same kind of creative satisfaction that their counterparts of a century before had derived from quilting. Consider the recipe for Gammy's Broken Glass Torte. It involves making separate pans of three Jell-O colors, cubing the gelatin, mixing the cubes with pineapple juice and whipped cream, pouring it all into a graham-cracker crust, chilling it, then slicing and serving it to oohs and aahs (and, presumably, grandchildren).

Of course, as anyone who has ever been hospitalized knows, unadulterated Jell-O is also standard sickroom fare. My colleague Patricia Sharpe recalls that, when she was little, "if I was peaked, Mother would whip up a batch. To this day, if I'm flu-ish or off my feed, I make Jell-O." Frankly, I was taken aback by this remark, as Pat, *Texas Monthly*'s food editor, has the most refined culinary sensibilities of any native Texan I know. But she went on to explain, "I don't even have to eat it, and I feel better."

This, I think, is how many people of my generation feel about Jell-O. We have fond memories of it, but not too many of us actually eat it anymore. Certainly our strict vegetarian members don't, since it is, after all, an animal byproduct. And the slogan "J-E-L-L-O," which dates back to 1934, has yielded to one that acknowledges the nation's eating-light obsession: "There's always room for Jell-O." But today Jell-O is much more than mere food. My kids know it mainly as a source of entertainment; when they were small, we used molds to make Jell-O Easter eggs (they bounce!). Teenagers eat it to help their nails grow long, or make a paste of it to temporarily dye their hair. Some diners use it as a vehicle for mounds of whipped cream (or faux-dairy Cool Whip, also a product of Jell-O's megacorp owner, Kraft Foods). A few folks have dived into giant vats of Jell-O; many more mix it with liquor and down it half-gelled as shots. And the stuff is a veteran performer: It has appeared in everything from Tom and Jerry cartoons to *Seinfeld* episodes. There's the scene in *National Lampoon's Christmas Vacation* involving Aunt Bethany, green Jell-O, and cat food, and—less famous but my favorite—the snippet in *Dancer, Texas Pop. 81* in which every elderly widow in town visits the hamlet's most eligible old bachelor, each bearing a container of homemade congealed this or that.

One of those containers surely holds Lime Jell-O Surprise. This deceptively pretty dish—you know, that mint-green slab that's a standard consolation casserole—may be beloved of bluehairs, but it will always be feared by small fry. For one thing, despite its candy color, its ingredients include vinegar and salt, so it treads dangerously close to aspic territory. Also, the recipe calls for cottage cheese, which renders the Jell-O opaque and hides various unwelcome ingredients (hence the "surprise" in the name). I remember my first bite of my aunt Merle's version, which I quickly relocated to my napkin; my taste buds screamed, "Not sweet!" and then, "Even worse!" as I bit into a piece of pimiento, which lurked in my serving along with celery and carrots—and pecans. When it comes to Texas cooking, there's always room for pecans.

*June 2004*

# LET ME CALL YOU SWEET-TART

ANNE DINGUS

If you're lucky, you'll find an old-fashioned soda fountain that will make you a cherry lime. It will make your summer day.

IT WAS A TYPICAL TEXAS SUMMER MORNING—sun shining, birds singing, people melting—when I ran into a young friend at the farmers' market. She was clutching that essential seasonal accessory, a cold canned drink, which happened to be one of the industry's timid forays into fusion, Coca-Cola with lime. "A lime Coke!" I said. "I drank a few of those in my day." She frowned prettily at me across the string beans and cream peas and said, "But . . . they just came out."

Actually, little missy, that particular American potable evolved about a hundred years ago. Back in the Dork Ages, a lime Coke (or a cherry-vanilla Dr Pepper or a strawberry lemonade) didn't come in a handy can. It was prepared on the spot at a soda fountain or a drive-in, with carbonated water and flavored syrup. Comparing the lime Coke of today with the sublime Coke I recall from, say, 1965 is like equating beef jerky with pit barbecue.

Whew! It's thirsty work standing on a soapbox! And to be honest, the lime Coke doesn't even top my list of favorite beverages (alcohol-free division). The soft drink with which I've had a lifelong *affaire de coeur*—and taste buds—is the cherry lime, a blend of cherry syrup, fizzy water, and fresh lime juice. It's sweet and tart and utterly ambrosial, and it's disappearing from Texas.

Anne
Dingus

The cherry lime evolved from the gin rickey, an early highball
supposedly named after Joe Rickey, a Washington lobbyist in the
late 1890s who became the nation's first major importer of limes.
The drink was an instant hit, and various bottlers promptly came
up with a soft version for teetotalers and tots, all under the generic label "rickey." By the twenties, when a gleaming chrome-and-
tile soda fountain was as indispensable to a town as a post office,
the cherry lime was as common as a Starbucks latte is today.

If properly made, a cherry lime is unusual among soft drinks
in that it is not only sweet and flavorful but also thirst quench-
ing. These attributes make it ideal for summertime refreshment
and explain why, like Brooklyn's egg cream, such a retro potion re-
tains a loyal following despite its elusive nature. In particular, the
cherry lime keeps hanging on in West Texas and the Panhandle.
I can think of several reasons why: Maybe workingmen such as
cowboys and roughnecks, who always need water and want sugar,
have kept the drink popular; the cheerful pink-and-green color
combo has always contrasted pleasantly with the sepia landscape;
and tradition surely plays a part (I'm a third-generation cherry-
limer). For us baby boomers, there was also the nutritional benefit. Just as sailors in the eighteenth century drank lime juice to
prevent scurvy on long sea voyages, so Panhandle kids during the
fifties and sixties depended on cherry limes to keep them healthy
and hap—hahahahaha. Sorry, just couldn't keep that up.

I'm of an age at which I can claim friends who are former soda
jerks. One is my colleague Gary Cartwright, who, before becoming a famous writer and general rapscallion, earned pin money
at Terry Brothers' Drug Store, in Arlington. "If I had a dime for
every cherry lime I made, I'd be in jail for fraud," he says. "They
only cost a nickel! As I recall, you filled a small Coke glass with
ice, added a squirt of plain syrup and a squirt of cherry, filled it
with carbonated water, and then squeezed in half a fresh lime."
That was back in the late forties, when Gary was a teenager, and
the formula hasn't changed a whit. My friend Hope Rodriguez
still recites the same recipe, which she prepared hundreds of times
at the Woolworth's lunch counter in downtown Austin 48 years
ago. But at home, her family devised an inexpensive cherry-lime
knockoff: "We mixed cherry Kool-Aid with fresh lime juice and

extra sugar. I was the third of ten kids, so we had to make every penny count."

When I was growing up in Pampa, the parched of throat could find a cherry lime at every burger joint, roadhouse, and cafe. My hometown is still, by modern standards, a cherry-lime stronghold. The best-ever purveyor: Jay's Drive-Inn. The employees have always been easygoing, efficient women who negotiate the tiny shack with a smooth choreography that suggests years of working around other bodies (and vats of hot grease). Almost everything on the menu is "frad"—burritos, hot dogs, jalapeños—except for the ice cream and drinks. For close to half a century, Jay's has set the bar for the cherry lime. For one thing, its mixologists distinguish between the cherry lime and the cherry limeade: The former is carbonated, the latter is not. For another, they don't add a maraschino cherry, for which I thank them. I confess a deep and abiding scorn for the maraschino cherry, which not only tastes like kiddie cough syrup but also reminds me of fruit cocktail, a fallback insta-salad my generation faced at dinner at least once a week. (A typical can contained only two cherry halves, sparking fights in any family with three or more kids.) The "m" cherry is just one reason I disdain the slapdash cherry lime prepared at Sonic, the only major fast-foodery in Texas that boasts the drink on its menu. Sonic's ersatz version also calls for Sprite and grenadine. (Bear in mind, the chain is headquartered in Oklahoma.) I assure you, though, that the servers at many small-town Dairy Queens or mom-and-pop joints remember the cherry lime. Even if it's not listed, ask—you just might get lucky.

Polling friends and colleagues for this story, I was amazed at how many had never had—or even heard of—a cherry lime. Inevitably these folks are city slickers, whose more sophisticated environs gave them access to an impressive assortment of ready-made drinks. But no manufacturer has ever successfully bottled or canned the cherry lime. Few have tried and one has frozen: Pepsi once tested a cherry-lime version of Slice; IBC, of root beer fame, sells cherry lime in a six-pack, but it's severely undercitrus'd; and in the seventies 7-Eleven offered the sweet-and-sour blend in a pretty darn decent tasting Slurpee.

At times, of course—church picnics, family reunions, road

trips—bottled drinks are a necessity. So let's raise a glass to a few of our state's favorite soda pops. Consider Dr Pepper, which was invented in Waco in 1885 and thus ranks as Texas's grand old brand. When I was little, kids thought Dr Pepper, with its cola-meets-fruit taste, contained prune juice (an urban legend that persists to this day). My friend Liz Aston had a more original theory while growing up in Angleton: "We all thought Dr Pepper tasted like what ants would taste like." What did Liz and I know? Today Dr Pepper is the nation's seventh-best-selling soft drink, with half a billion cases swigged in 2004. Liz is, however, a proponent of another venerable Texas beverage: Big Red, which was also invented in Waco, although a mere 68 years ago. Big Red is a fixture at Juneteenth celebrations and backyard barbecues and has a taste that defies description: Cherry? Strawberry? Liquefied Bazooka? "Once we got into surfing, Big Red was the drink of choice," Liz says. "I think that because it was so candylike, it went well with the salt water. I still want Big Red every time I go to the beach."

Many of Texas's indie soft drinks quickly hit hard times, but one survivor is Delaware Punch, which dates back to 1913, when its secret formula included such then-exotic juices as pineapple and passion fruit. The origin of the name is a mystery, as it was invented in San Antonio. (Then again, Texas Punch was bottled in Pennsylvania. Perhaps the pop is always pinker in the other state.) Lovers of grape-flavored soda had bunches to pick from, but Grapette was the coolest, and not just because it actually tasted like grape juice. It was famous for its artsy bottles; one featured multicolored polka dots, and another had a raised "twisted" pattern that made it recognizable by feel when a thirsty patron was attempting to remove a bottle from one of those giant floor coolers full of arm-numbing slush. (Note to the nostalgic: Plant a Texas mountain laurel in your yard. The blossoms smell a lot like Grapette.) And does anyone else remember Pommac? It was a sparkling apple-flavored drink—Swedish, believe it or not—that enjoyed a brief Texas fling in the sixties. By then most of the state's original brands—such as San Antonio's fruit-flavored Hippo sodas, so called because they were extrabig (sixteen ounces) and touted the city's zoo—had fizzled out, left flat by the likes of Coca-Cola and other beverage behemoths.

And if you ask me, little missy, most of them weren't worth a sip. Give me a cherry lime any day. May it live on in Pampa and Tahoka, Conway and Odessa, and other points west. I'll drink 'em as long as I can find 'em—just as I have since I was Nehi to a grasshopper.

*August 2005*

# PERSONALITIES

# PIT SPLIT

JOE NICK PATOSKI

How a family beef could spell the end of one of the state's best barbecue joints.

ON THE SURFACE, it's little more than a tenant-landlord dispute aggravated by the fact that the renter and the owner happen to be brother and sister, respectively. But when the business is Kreuz Market in Lockhart, a storied establishment that dates back to around 1900 and is frequently cited as the best barbecue joint in the free world, the disagreement might as well be a declaration of war.

It all began in 1990, the year Edgar "Smitty" Schmidt, Kreuz's owner, passed away. Schmidt, who had bought it from Alvin Kreuz and two other co-owners in 1948, sold the business to his sons, Rick and Don, but bequeathed the building and the property it occupied to his daughter, Nina Sells. ("Why he did it that way, he's the only one who can speculate," Rick says.) Rick was raised in the market, and Nina worked there part-time until 1983 (she is now in her fourth term as the county clerk for Caldwell County). Rick, his two sons, and Don have continued operating Kreuz the same as always, serving smoked meats straight from the pits on pieces of butcher paper, with no forks, no sauces, and no side dishes. But that will officially end on August 31, when their lease with Nina expires. Rick says that he wants to renew it and extend the current five-year option but that his sister wants to raise the rent to $400,000 over five years, a figure he calls "exorbitant." She says she has tried to be reasonable but has been unable to come to terms with her brother. Negotiations became so contentious that Rick and Nina each hired lawyers, and media attention by the *Austin American-Statesman* and CBS's *Eye on America* only fanned the flames.

How could it come to this? Blame it on a volatile combination of business and family. "We don't have an inheritance problem," Rick contends. "We have a landlady problem. I was trying to make a deal with my sister. I wanted to buy the property. She kept telling me it wasn't for sale. I'd at least like an option to lease for another twenty years, but she said no to that. I looked her in the eye and asked, 'Why?' She looked at me and said, 'You think I couldn't run a barbecue place?'"

"My customers are really upset about it," Rick says, noting that business has picked up considerably because of a steady stream of pilgrimages from faithful out-of-town customers who fear the end is near. "Some of them are mad at me. I've heard she's been getting hate mail. It's not something you're proud of when you don't get along with your family, but it's not a family squabble. It's business."

Nina hardly deserves the evil landlord stereotype. A demure, soft-spoken blonde, she says the events of the past year and a half have driven her to tears on several occasions. Other than a vague allusion to past family problems, she says she doesn't want to dwell on the particulars. "It's emotional when it's family," she says. Nina says that she met with her brother in late 1997 to discuss repairs. "Rick wanted improvements," she says, "and I wasn't necessarily against it." He wanted to build a new dining room; she was most concerned about repairs to the existing building. "I felt like we had seven years left in the option to make the repairs, but if we couldn't agree to do it by then, I didn't want to extend the lease for twenty years," Nina says. What she describes as the "double the rent article" in the *American-Statesman* last April, which she believes made her sound inflexible, hardened her position. "In a way, it became 'Sell or Move.' It was more of an ultimatum, and it's hard to negotiate that way."

"That was the icing on the cake," says Nina's husband, Jim

Sells, a teacher at Lockhart High School for the past 22 years. It turns out that Nina wasn't just blowing smoke when she later announced her intention to open a new barbecue restaurant and meat market in the building she owns: Her husband is part of a cooking team whose beef brisket has earned first-place awards at Lockhart's Chisholm Trail Cookoff the past two years, and her husband and her two sons, John and James Fullilove, all walked away with blue ribbons at cook-offs in Luling and Lubbock last year. The new place, she says, will be called Smitty's.

As for Rick, he promises more room and more comfort at a new Kreuz's just four tenths of a mile north of the present location—plans that were part of his desire to improve the old market before negotiations fell apart. "We're going to use a lot of brick, a lot of metal, and a lot of wood," he says. "It's not going to be fancy. It's not going to be pretty. But I'm not going to build a phony place. Customers will be close to the fire but not blistered by it the way they are now." Rick is also doubling the number of cooking pits and upgrading them with quarter-inch steel lining instead of the sheet metal currently used. "The new ones are going to outlive me," he says. "I've already built a prototype and tested it on thirty-five of my beer-drinking friends, who are real critical. I burst a lot of bubbles because they said it tasted like it came from here, so I'm real confident the quality can be maintained. I'm gonna try to maintain one hundred percent of what I've got here. Roy, my pit man, even wants to drag a ceremonial bucket of coals from here to the new place."

Less certain is whether Rick can maintain the unique atmosphere of Kreuz's. "We're losing a tradition and the memories that go with it," he admits. Then again, change is a constant, even in a family operation as traditional as this one. After all, Kreuz's became the Schmidts' place after the Kreuz heirs decided they didn't want to run it. Furthermore, half of Kreuz's current dining area didn't exist until 1979, when the business expanded. "A lot of people have misconceptions that it's always been here like this and never changed," Rick says.

The upside of the pit split is that Lockhart could soon be home to four world-class BBQ places (in "Smokin'!," *Texas Monthly*'s May 1997 ranking of the state's best barbecue joints, Lockhart was the only town that had three: Kreuz's, Black's Barbecue, and Chisholm Trail B-B-Q). That's a prospect Nina Sells believes in. "We think it can happen," she says. "Otherwise we wouldn't be doing it." The downside is the possibility that neither Smitty's nor the new Kreuz's will rate with the original. Certainly Kreuz's competitors are hoping the barbecue battle continues to be a distraction. The owners of Black's, whose motto is "Oldest in Texas, Same Family," have placed portable signs on U.S. 183 that read, "No Crisis Here" and "No Feud, Just Good Food."

All of which leaves Rick to ponder what Smitty would make of this if he were alive. "He wouldn't be happy of hearing about the market moving," he insists. "I know that."

*February 1999*

# TEXAS FOOD CONQUERS THE WORLD

PATRICIA SHARPE

From Riyadh to the Rio Grande, Southwestern cuisine is sweeping the globe, thanks to the skill—and salesmanship—of a group of ambitious Texas chefs.

IT WAS TWO SUMMERS ago in Ann Arbor, as I stood on State Street, staring at a menu taped in the front window of the Red Hawk Bar and Grill, that the full force of the realization struck me. Listed there among the usual soups, sandwiches, and pasta salads were—crab cakes grilled with red and green chiles in red *mole* sauce. Here I was in Michigan, home of—well, I'm not sure what, but definitely not *mole* sauce—and I could walk into a restaurant and order as if I were in Dallas or Houston. A dozen years ago, this would not have happened. A dozen years ago, Southwestern cuisine barely had a name. To the degree it existed at all, it was a glint in the eyes of a handful of young chefs in Texas (plus a couple in California) who were holed up in their kitchens inventing amazing new things to do with jicama and habaneros. Today the culinary craze that started in the Lone Star State is a national, indeed, an international phenomenon.

There was a time, and it wasn't that long ago, when cilantro was just a weird Mexican herb. When a chile relleno was a bell pepper stuffed with spiced hamburger meat. Now, the popular Zagat restaurant guides routinely include a category for "Southwestern." In March Dallas's KERA will air the pilot of a potential thirteen-part public television series by Dallas chef Stephan Pyles on his style of Southwestern cooking—and this, mind you, comes hard on the heels of PBS's *Southwestern Supper* by *Moosewood Cookbook* author Mollie Katzen. The Great Southwest Cuisine Catalog mails out 40,000 to 50,000 copies a year hyping its salsas, turkey chorizo, and piñon brittle. Last year a United Airlines in-flight video featured Dallas's Southwestern virtuoso Dean Fearing as one of the top reasons to visit the city. In October the Hotel Al Khozama in Riyadh held a Southwestern food festival. In its winter 1996 catalog, the William Morrow publishing company announced three new cookbooks on "the cornerstones of Southwestern cuisine." Santa Fe's Coyote Cafe chef and owner, Mark Miller, reports that his cookbooks are selling like tortilla chips in, among other places, Australia. Not only that, the peripatetic Miller is now massaging a deal to do Coyote Cafe spin-offs in Singapore and Kuala Lumpur.

Southwestern cuisine is everywhere. Even restaurants with other national affiliations will slip a little tequila-marinated salmon or ancho linguine onto the menu, or use "Southwestern" as a buzzword to hype dishes that have precious little to do with the genre. It all made me wonder, how did the real thing actually start, and how did it become a national rage? And so it was that last November I found myself once again standing in front of a building, except this one was not in Ann Arbor but in Dallas, on University Avenue. The edifice was a generic duplex of orangy-brown brick with fifties-style casement windows, and yet in a way it was a historic building because it was here that the idea for Southwestern cuisine was born, or perhaps I should say hatched.

Beside me in the circular driveway was Anne Greer, a petite, energetic blonde in a red blazer, spotless white turtleneck, and black-and-white-checked skirt. A cookbook author and restaurant consultant who seems to operate on perpetual fast forward, Greer lived in this house in the eighties, and as the five o'clock traffic swirled past us, she told me, "This is where we met. We would have dinner out back by the grill and then we'd plot about how to get people to *notice* us."

The "we" that Greer referred to was herself and a loosely knit group of six other young Texas chefs, and the bond that united them was the realization that each, in his or her own restaurant or hotel kitchen, was doing something exciting and very new with Texas food. "We started meeting in about 1984 because I could see that we were all doing something similar," Greer told me later over ceviche at Cafe Pacific as we leafed through her file of old clippings, "and we wanted to get the word out about it."

The group that came together at Greer's and several other homes over the next few months read, in part, like a future who's who of Southwestern cuisine. Five of the participants were from Dallas: Greer, then 40, was a consultant for the Loews Anatole Hotel and the author of *The Cuisine of the American Southwest*. Dean Fearing, 29, was the chef at the Anatole's Verandah Club. Kevin Hopkins, 30, headed the Anatole's Nana Grill. Avner Samuel, 28, was in charge of the restaurant at the Mansion on Turtle Creek hotel. Stephan Pyles, 32, was the chef and co-owner of Routh Street Cafe. The other two attendees were from Houston: Robert Del Grande, 29, was the chef at Cafe Annie, and Amy Ferguson, 28, was at Charley's 517.

The meetings centered on dinner, a kind of glorified potluck at which all the dishes were fabulous because all the cooks were pros. The seven of them ate what they had brought, hoping to impress each other, and traded tips, but mainly they schemed and plotted ways to get attention. They knew each other only vaguely, but they had traits in common that were to prove the foundation of the nascent cuisine. They were roughly the same age, they all had classical training, and they all were fascinated and inspired by Mexican food. They knew *The Cuisines of Mexico* by Diana Kennedy, and some of them had taken her classes. Indeed, the influence of the feisty ex-Brit on the Southwestern phenomenon cannot be overestimated. In the lessons she gave across the country and in the harangues she delivered on authenticity and purity, she paved the way for a generation of cooks. Even though the newcomers' riffs on Mexican cuisine overstepped what Kennedy deemed acceptable, she was the one who showed them that there was life beyond the No. 2 Dinner.

The eighties were, moreover, a time of tremendous ferment in the culinary world. In France nouvelle cuisine had dethroned, or at least shaken up, that country's classical cuisine, and in America, the so-called new American cuisine was bringing to regional dishes all over the country a respect that they had never before enjoyed. Heretofore, "serious" restaurants had served a stuffy, vaguely European repertoire known as continental cuisine. But with the rise of regionalism, suddenly it was not only acceptable but chic to put biscuits, smoked pork, cheese grits, and absolutely anything with pomegranate seeds on the menu.

Given their backgrounds and the heady climate of experimentation, it was almost inevitable that this group of ambitious young professionals should turn to Texas dishes. Why couldn't French methods be married to the traditions of Mexico and Texas? Suppose you added a purée of ancho chiles to a classic demi-glace? Why not take a corn husk and make a tamale of rice pudding with *crème anglaise*? The only possible answer to these questions was another question: Why not?

As Greer and I finished lunch, she passed me a yellowing photograph from the August 5, 1984, *Dallas Times Herald* showing the gang of seven lined up behind a table, looking like a bunch of baby boomers at a suburban dinner party. It was surprising to see, in retrospect, how un-Southwestern the table appeared, with its white china and sedate presentations. Similarly, the story, by Michael Bauer, shows a trend still in its infancy. Bauer wrote, "Greer dabbed oil on her hands to protect them from the [jalapeños]. The technique was new to Ferguson, who appreciated the tip." But the menu he described—swordfish in achiote, grilled corn salad with poblanos and cilantro—was already getting with the program.

All told, the Algonquin Round Table of Texas cooking met perhaps half a dozen times. Greer, who had a natural instinct for public relations, took the lead and engineered a number of events. It was she, for instance, who saw to it that Bauer was invited to dinner, and the series of three articles that he subsequently wrote were some of the earliest to recognize what was happening. In fact, the name "new Southwestern cuisine" seems to have been first used in print on August 7, 1983, in a story that Bauer wrote on Greer.

Over the next several months and years, the group—collectively and individually—cooked for anyone who would do a story. As newspaper food sections and magazines chronicled the spread of Southwestern cuisine, it became apparent that the idea had simultaneously occurred on the West Coast, where John Sedlar (then at Saint Estèphe in Manhattan Beach, California) and Mark Miller (then at the Fourth Street Grill in Berkeley) were serving jazzed-up posole and blue-cornmeal dessert crêpes to flocks of customers. This both reassured and spurred the Texans on. They got themselves invited to entertain food writers like Ellen Brown of *USA Today*, and they asked famous chefs like Jean-Louis Palladin to come see what they were doing. In October 1984 Marian Burros, the well-known *New York Times* food writer, was interviewed by a local magazine, in which she said of Dallas restaurants, "There's a real revolution going on" with the emerging Southwestern cooking. *Times* restaurant critic Craig Claiborne heaped praise on Pyles and Fearing. In a major coup in 1985, the Mansion hosted the American Institute of Food and Wine's dinner honoring Julia Child, at which the menu included whole catfish and blue-corn tamales. The Mansion's waiters were horrified at what they were asked to serve the grande dame of cooking in America, but Child loved it.

Of all the activities that garnered national recognition, though, one of the most significant was the Hill Country Wine and Food Festival. Started in 1986 by Ed and Susan Auler, the owners of Fall Creek Vineyards, the festival grew in a matter of three years to be a major American food event. Wine and food professionals from all over descended on Austin each spring, where they attended seminars and took time out for creative lunches prepared by, among others, Del Grande, Fearing, Pyles, and Greer. The press took to calling the four young cooks the "Texas mafia," a name that fit their friendship and single-minded focus.

The final ingredient that boosted Southwestern cuisine onto the national stage was oil—not the extra-virgin stuff but Texas crude. The oil boom of the early eighties not only provided legions of Texans with disposable cash but filled grocery and specialty stores everywhere with exotic imported foodstuffs from Mexico, Europe, and Asia. The boom also fostered an attitude conducive to creativity. Dean Fearing, who has observed Dallas in high times and low from his vantage point at the glitzy Mansion on Turtle Creek, says, "When the economy is good, your customers are open to new things. When they have expendable money, they're willing to experiment." Judged by this yardstick, the eighties were exactly the right time to launch a daring and unproven culinary style.

It has now been twelve years since Southwestern cuisine began. Of the original group who plotted around Anne Greer's grill, four have kept in touch with the Southwestern style but basically moved in other directions. Amy Ferguson relocated to Hawaii. Kevin Hopkins is a partner in a Dallas Thai restaurant, Toy's Cafe. Avner Samuel is at the Landmark restaurant at the Melrose Hotel in Dallas, cooking in a "global eclectic" style that incorporates Southwestern influences. Greer dropped out of sight for several years to care for her son after a devastating car accident. These days she does restaurant consulting and is planning another Southwestern cookbook. As for the other three mafiosi—Pyles, Fearing, and Del Grande—they have ridden the movement to national culinary stardom and beyond.

Southwestern cuisine is now a mature master, an elder statesman. It has created its own classics, including jicama slaw, cilantro pesto, tomatillo-poblano sauce, roasted-corn salad, mango pico, and more. It has also been copied far and wide, though not always with integrity. As Pyles says, "In the past five or six years this whole style has filtered down into restaurants that are certainly more approachable and less expensive than ours. Restaurants like Chili's and Bennigan's all serve something that screams 'Southwestern cuisine.'" Which is why the Texas trio are at pains to put some distance between themselves and the mainstream, dumbed-down versions that populate mid-level eateries all over the country.

They are also at pains to emphasize that they have moved forward and expanded their repertoires. Del Grande jokes, "I look at older menus—tamales-stuffed-with-achiote-shrimp-and-ancho-poblano-jalapeño-serrano-*mole*—and they seem like a cartoon." Of the three, his style remains the most Mexican and rustic, but over the years it has softened and become more subtle, with multinational highlights. Fearing's style has taken off in Asian, Middle Eastern, and North African directions. And Pyles has developed what he calls the New Texas cuisine, with sophisticated spins on traditional Southern, Mexican, cowboy, and Cajun dishes.

Southwestern cuisine has been very good to Texas. The state's romantic, rough-hewn image provided a ready-made backdrop for the movement, while the style's finesse dazzled critics, who never expected such refinement from the land of cactus and Cadillacs. It trained a national spotlight on the state, and over the years it has done as much to raise the status of Texas culture as have institutions like the Kimbell Art Museum and the Houston Grand Opera. Southwestern cuisine has permeated the country like mesquite smoke, but as Fearing says, "One of the most marvelous things about that whole explosion is that everyone's eyes are still on Texas." If you want the real thing, you still have to come here to get it.

*February 1996*

# CONFESSIONS OF A
# SKINNY BITCH

PATRICIA SHARPE

Over the past thirty years, as a restaurant reviewer and an editor for this magazine, I've had my share of flaccid flautas, gummy grits, and barely edible brisket—and some pretty extraordinary meals as well. Yes, it's nice getting paid to eat out. No, it's not always as much fun as it sounds. Yes, it's a struggle to stay this thin. Any more questions?

THE EXCHANGE GOES SOMETHING LIKE THIS. I'm chit-chatting with people I've met at a party, and the subject of jobs comes up. My new acquaintances turn out to be artists, computer geeks, hippo trainers, whatever. I confess that I'm a restaurant reviewer. There's a short pause while they look me up and down as if I were a two-headed poodle at the Westminster dog show. Then someone says, with more than a touch of resentment, "*Soooo,* if you eat out for a living, how come you're so thin?" And right off the bat, they're mad at me. It's not just strangers, either. Two of my dear friends have taken to calling me "that skinny bitch." To which I say, "Guilty as charged."

Last December 1 I celebrated thirty years at this magazine. That's a lot of crème brûlée under the bridge, folks. During that time, food fads have risen (fajitas and Southwestern cuisine) and fallen (blackened redfish), and once-fabled Texas restaurants have vanished like a snow cone on the Fourth of July (how many of you remember Mr. Peppe, in Dallas, or the original Naples on Broadway, in San Antonio, or Che, in Houston?). Texas has changed

*Patricia*
*Sharpe*

from a state that eats at home to one that eats out, and Dallas and Houston have taken their places on the national culinary stage. Since it was founded, in 1973, this magazine has published more than 28,000 restaurant reviews. If that indicates anything, it's that people are endlessly fascinated with food and dining. And judging by the queries I get, they're also curious about the arcane practice of restaurant reviewing. So I thought this might be as good a time as any to answer a question or two, including the inevitable . . .

*How do you stay so thin?*

The answer is really, really simple: I'm neurotic. I eat only half of what I'm served, and if I do gain a pound, I freak out and take it off immediately. (For the record, I am five feet seven inches tall and weigh 117 pounds.) My weight-loss system is a slightly twisted version of the South Beach Diet: I don't eat anything white. All right, that's an exaggeration, but I do eat very little sugar, bread, pasta, potatoes, or rice (including, alas, risotto). And I watch the butter and cheese. Occasionally, I have to admit, I overdo this regimen and end up famished at odd times, so I always carry stashes of almonds and Southwest Airlines peanuts in my briefcase. As for the next inevitable question—"Do you exercise?"—the answer is not a lot; I walk a mile and a half a day. Does sticking to a diet make it hard to evaluate a meal? Absolutely not. All you do is pay attention and savor each bite.

*What is the reaction when your plate goes back to the kitchen half-full?*

Uneaten food terrifies restaurants, because most people in our society, especially men, clean their plates. Their mothers have guilt-tripped them with stories of starving orphans in far-flung lands. This is one reason among many that ours is a nation of fatties, but I digress. Frequently, waiters ask me if something was wrong. I just say I wasn't very hungry. Sometimes they persist—"Are you sure?"—which is really, really annoying. If I don't want a hassle or if I worry about hurting the cook's feelings at a small place, I ask for a doggie bag. And I always get a doggie bag when I'm eating five or six meals a day for a story like "Pit Stops," our barbecue roundup in the May 2003 issue. If I can find a homeless person to give the food to, I do; if I'm on the road, the leftovers end up at my motel. More than once I've left half a dozen to-go boxes stacked beside the bed. God knows what the maids thought.

*Did your family love to cook?*

No, just the opposite. When I was growing up in the fifties, Texas was a vast Middle American wasteland of overcooked hamburger steaks, waterlogged peas and carrots, Jell-O salads, and TV dinners, the latter of which we ate—I swear to God—on folding metal tables while sitting in front of the television set watching *Your Hit Parade* and *Gunsmoke*. On top of this, my mother was a protofeminist who embraced the liberating notion that a woman's place was *not* in the kitchen. Thus, she never used a fresh vegetable if she could get her hands on a canned or frozen one, and she had an absolute love affair with instant mashed potatoes. Oh, Mother could cook if she wanted to: Her lemon chiffon pie was divine, and I loved her vegetable soup. But she preferred to spend her time reading Thomas Wolfe's *Look Homeward, Angel* rather than slaving over a hot stove. Her weekly canned-salmon croquettes were one reason I adored eating in restaurants. They served gorgeous food that I never saw at home, plus they were exciting and grown-up. The fact that we couldn't afford to eat out much made them even more alluring. Restaurants were like movies to me, an escape from humdrum real life and, shudder, real food.

*Have you always been interested in food?*

If you had told my parents I would one day be a restaurant critic, they would have fallen on the floor laughing. My childhood food quirks were a major pain in the posterior. I was the kid who had to be removed from nursery school because I refused to consume the vile lunches they served (asphaltlike fried liver and slimy okra with tomatoes). I was the one who pitched a fit if a sandwich had been cut into squares instead of triangles. I hardly ate during the first grade except for drinking gallons of milk. I remember one little boy saying to me, in a thick Southern drawl, "Pa-*tree*-sha, why are you so *skinnn*-ny?" The answer is that there wasn't a lot of food to like back then. The turning point, for me, was marrying a man who loved to cook. My husband was only 22, but he wowed our circle of friends by using real butter, not margarine, and making chocolate cake *and* icing from scratch, not a mix. One time we gave a dinner party, and he rolled veal around homemade stuffing to make "veal birds." He knew how to make Danish pastries filled with marzipan. This was the true beginning of my infatuation with food.

*How did you get to be a restaurant reviewer?*

Honestly, I fell into this job like it was a tub of butter. I started out proofreading the magazine's restaurant reviews and calendar of events, plus answering the phones and running errands. I could have continued being a gofer for years, but fortunately, then–senior editor Griffin Smith decided he wanted to write features full-time. As a result, I inherited his job of editing the restaurant guide. What I knew about food in 1975 could have been put in a demitasse spoon, but I did love to eat. Bill Broyles, the magazine's founding editor, said, "Learn everything you can, take cooking lessons, go to the best places—we'll pay for it." So I did. One memorable summer, a friend and I went to five Michelin two- and three-star restaurants in France in one week, including the legendary Le Pyramide. Foie gras and truffles were our crack cocaine. Looking back, I was in the right place at the right time. Texas was awakening to the joys of fine food, and we all rode that wave into shore together. Lucky me, I'm still riding it today.

*How do you review a restaurant?*

When I put a bite of food in my mouth, I unconsciously give it a grade: A through F. The A's are the easiest—those are pure, intense pleasure, like Dallas restaurant Aurora's famous amuse-bouche, a dab of warm vanilla custard shot through with the earthy flavor of black truffles and topped with maple whipped cream. The F's are easy too—they are off, discordant, like fingernails on a blackboard; imagine foie gras blended with white chocolate, a dish I've actually had. The hardest are the C's, because nothing stands out—they're just there, neither wonderful nor awful. While the sensation is still fresh, I open my little spiral-bound notebook and jot down words to jog my memory: "The risotto would have made excellent library paste." Not every restaurant critic takes notes, but I taste so much food it's easy to forget the details. Over the years, I've tried everything from using a tiny hand-held recorder to calling the office on my cell phone and leaving whispered messages ("The profiteroles were like golf balls"). But I always come back to paper. Sometimes the waiters notice the notebook, but by the time the food is on the table, it's too late to change it. When I get home, or back to the hotel, I type up my thoughts on everything: food, service, decor. If a dish has a lot of ingredients or is just hard to get a handle on, I'll get a doggie bag and examine it later (but I don't retaste anything that's not fresh).

### Do you eat alone?

I almost always ask one to three people to eat with me, occasionally more. And I always eat off their plates (or have them pass me samples). My favorite eaters are the ones who'll deconstruct the details with me—"Do you think that's anise or tarragon?"—and offer their own insights. The ones who drive me crazy never go beyond "That's fabulous" or "That sucks" and yammer nonstop about their daughter's trailer-trash boyfriend or their mother's bile duct operation while I'm trying to take notes, not to mention enjoy the food.

### How do you decide what to order?

If I'm doing a review of a familiar restaurant, I might sample as few as two entrées, with sides, plus an appetizer or a dessert. If the place is new to me and has a complex menu, I go several times and try at least five entrées. The first thing I turn to is the list of specialties of the house; I want to see what the chef considers his signature dishes and strong points. After that, I look for anything creative or slightly unusual, say, duck breast with truffled pears and a juniper-port reduction. Sirloin with Roquefort butter may be delicious, but it's hardly the latest thing. On the other hand, a dish doesn't *have* to be creative to impress me, especially at places

*Patricia*    serving a traditional and moderately priced cuisine, like Mexican
*Sharpe*    or Middle Eastern. But the higher the prices, the more I want
something that sends me somewhere I've never been before.

*Who pays for the food?*

The magazine pays for the food, of course. That's the way all legitimate publications operate; no freebies allowed.

*Do you wear disguises?*

Sorry to disappoint you, but I have no Carol Channing wigs,
Grand Ole Opry hats, or Anna Wintour sunglasses in my closet.
I don't wear a disguise, nor do any of the dozen restaurant reviewers I know at other publications. Disguises are mainly a *New York
Times* and *Washington Post* phenomenon, because mug shots of
those singularly powerful critics are tacked up in restaurant kitchens all over the two cities. On the other hand, I (and all professional reviewers) prefer to be anonymous, so I generally make reservations under an assumed name to keep the staff from making a
fuss over me. (Occasionally I forget which nom de cuisine I used,
which elicits some peculiar stares as I flounder around: "Um, see
if you have a 'Swartz.' No? Well, what about 'Smulyan'?")

Of course, sometimes I'm recognized, and that can be tricky.
Once, Tony's, in Houston, sent out a bottle of very expensive wine.
We solved that problem by not drinking any. But the worst episode was the time, many years ago, when the owner of a Chinese
restaurant in Austin appeared with a fine teapot and announced
that he wanted to give it to me. I tried to explain that I couldn't accept gifts. He cajoled. I insisted. He kept handing me the teapot. I
kept handing it back. Finally, at the end of the meal, I left it on the
table and my guest and I sneaked out the door. Just as we drove
away, he came running out with the teapot, looking baffled and
hurt. We could never bear to go back.

*Do you have to train to become a restaurant critic?*

No. It's just like being a movie, theater, or book reviewer; anybody can do it if she (or he) can persuade somebody to hire her.

Predictably, this drives chefs and restaurateurs up the wall; they rant about unqualified reviewers—but only when they get bad reviews. To them I say, with all due respect, "Fine. The day you decide that someone should pass a culinary exam before he can open a restaurant and charge money, then we'll discuss qualifying tests for reviewers." My own feeling is that in the end, journalistic Darwinism sorts it all out. On-target reviewers last and off-base ones don't, just as good restaurants thrive and bad ones close. The public is the final arbiter of taste.

*Do you write the reviews in* Texas Monthly's Dining Guide *every month?*

Yes, and at Christmas, eight tiny reindeer and I deliver presents to all the good little boys and girls in the entire world. Wait, I think I blacked out for a minute. In fact, the magazine has twenty freelance reviewers around the state, plus four staff people in Austin, who do the visits and write the copy. We stay busy: More than two hundred reviews a month are written, edited, and fact-checked for the eleven cities and six regions covered in the Dining Guide. I write at least a couple of reviews a month, and of course, when I do a feature story like last month's "Where to Eat Now 2005," I visit all those restaurants myself.

*Have you or your reviewers had any run-ins with chefs or restaurateurs?*

I've never been tossed out of a restaurant, but in the eighties our Austin reviewer (let's call the poor dear Jane Doe) came close. She was standing in the vestibule of a very nice restaurant when she was spotted by the owner, who had somehow found out who she was. In a voice so loud that the wineglasses rattled, he said, "Well, well, well, if it isn't Mrs. Doe. Are you the person who reviews for *Texas Monthly?*" She stammered that she wasn't, but he had made his point. "I'm *so* glad you aren't," he said, "because if you *were*, I would ask you to leave." She was a wreck the rest of the evening. The funniest incident happened in the seventies, when Emil Vogely, then the chef at Jeffrey's, in Austin, wrote me a scathing letter in which he demanded to know "whose ass you have to kiss or kick" to get a star from *Texas Monthly*. My reply, which I no longer remember, just fanned the flames, because he then stormed up to the office, where we proceeded to harangue each other for thirty minutes. When he said the magazine was being disrespectful by referring to him as Emil, not Chef Emil, I told him I would gladly call him Chef Emil if he addressed me as Editor Pat. (Afterward, everybody in the office took to calling me Editor Pat.) Later, Emil and I became friends, and we have laughed about that incident more than once. Thank God most chefs these days have PR agents, who trip them when they charge out the door to do battle with restaurant critics.

*What is the best thing you've ever eaten?*

Fraises des bois ("strawberries of the woods"). The first—and, sadly, only—time I had them was about twenty years ago, at Alain Chapel, a Michelin three-star restaurant near Lyon. My friend Chris Durden and I had eaten the most amazing meal, accompanied by many different wines, and when we finished, the waiter brought out a plate of fraises des bois as an after-dinner treat. They were bright red, fragrant, and so small I popped three in my mouth at once. Omigod. The flavor was like all of summer concentrated in one bite—strawberries from heaven. I'm sure my cheeks flushed; I think my brain waves changed. During those weeks in France, fraises des bois were one of many epiphanies about the sensual pleasures and possibilities of eating. I'm not sure that food is ever better than sex, but it can be pretty darn close.

*What is the worst thing you've ever eaten?*

Ant eggs with a pulque chaser. Actually, the ant eggs weren't bad. I had them at a charming, rustic hotel in the Mexican countryside near Puebla, where my friend Gini Garcia and I had gone to forage for mushrooms with two eccentric Canadians. At lunch, ant eggs were on the menu, an indigenous dish that has achieved some notoriety as part of the so-called Aztec cuisine. They looked like small grains of rice and were just about as bland. With enough pico de gallo, you could hardly taste them. The pulque, which is the viscous fermented sap of agave plants, was a different story.

Our Canadian guides tested it first and pronounced it "the best
we've ever had." All I can say is this: If you can imagine curdled
milk that has been boiled for hours with old gym socks and stinkbugs, you can imagine pulque. The texture was a cross between
saliva and mucus. And this pulque, mind you, was the good stuff.

*What's the worst service you've ever had?*

In "the customer is always wrong" category, the worst was at the
dining room of the long-gone Hotel Meridien, in Houston. Our
meal had been fantastic, and I ordered gâteau au chocolat for dessert. On a whim, I decided I wanted raspberry purée with it instead of the listed vanilla-bean crème anglaise. I had seen raspberry sauce on the menu, so I knew it was available. Our waiter, a
gray-haired Frenchman who obviously considered being in Texas
equivalent to being in the Australian outback, did *not* approve.
"No, madame," he said, "raspberry sauce is not correct." I told him,
"But I *like* raspberry sauce and chocolate." He looked at me like
I had been raised by wolves, so I added, "I've had chocolate and
raspberry at other places." He shook his finger at me like I was a
naughty schoolgirl and said, "No, no, *no!*" And that was that. I ate
crème anglaise, and he got a 5 percent tip.

*March 2005*

# TASTEMAKER OF THE
# CENTURY—HELEN CORBITT

 PRUDENCE MACKINTOSH

S he delivered us from canned fruit cocktail—and gave us confidence that the civilizing pleasures of the table were within our reach.

IN THE YEARS B.C. (BEFORE CORBITT), Texans had no artichokes, no fresh raspberries, no herbs except decorative parsley, only beef (chicken-fried, barbecued, or well-done), potatoes (fried or mashed and topped with a glop of cream gravy), and wedges of iceberg with sweet orange dressing. Fruit salad meant canned pears or pineapple with a dollop of mayonnaise and a grating of cheddar cheese. Canned asparagus was a remarked-upon delicacy, as were LeSueur canned peas. The introduction of the TV dinner in the fifties would be a step up for some households.

Into this bleak culinary landscape came a young Irish Catholic Yankee named Helen Corbitt. In a career that spanned nearly forty years in Texas, she delivered us from canned fruit cocktail, plates of fried brown food, and too much bourbon and branch into a world of airy soufflés, poached fish, chanterelle mushrooms, fresh salsify, Major Grey's Chutney, crisp steamed vegetables, and fine wine. She was a creative pioneer who came here reluctantly and learned to love us. She taught us, she fed us, she entertained us, and best of all, before she left us in 1978, she wrote down the how-to of Corbitt hospitality in five cookbooks, giving us confidence that the civilizing pleasures of the table were within our reach. Superstar chefs Dean Fearing, Stephan Pyles, and Robert

Del Grande may pay homage to Julia Child and Simone Beck, but long before they learned to clarify butter, there was Corbitt.

Helen Corbitt was born on January 25, 1906, in upstate New York into a home where good food was highly valued and generously shared. After her graduation from Skidmore College in Saratoga Springs, New York, with a degree in home economics, her plans for medical school were derailed by the Depression. She took a job as a therapeutic dietitian at Presbyterian Hospital in Newark, New Jersey, then went on to Cornell Medical Center in New York, where she persuaded doctors that sick people would respond more favorably to food if it was properly seasoned and attractively served.

In 1940 Corbitt was offered a job teaching catering and restaurant management at the University of Texas. "I said, 'Who the hell wants to go to Texas?'" she later told *Dallas Times Herald* reporter Julia Sweeney. "Only I didn't say 'hell' in those days. I learned to swear in Texas." Two weeks after she arrived in Austin, she was asked to do a dinner for a hotel convention using only Texas products: "What I thought of Texas products wasn't fit to print!" Like an alchemist, she transformed prosaic black-eyed peas for the dinner, adding some garlic, onion, vinegar, and oil and christening them "Texas Caviar." Neiman Marcus would later sell thousands of cans of the stuff. The University Tea Room, a lab she created for her classes in the U.T. Home Economics Building, became such a popular eating spot for faculty and students that it soon merited its own space near Twenty-fourth and San Jacinto. Corbitt left Austin for a more lucrative position at the Houston Country Club in 1942. She still wasn't sold on Texas and planned to stay just long enough to get on her feet and buy a ticket back to New York. She claimed that she didn't unpack her suitcase for the first six months. But after a year in Houston, she had decided to stay. "I was having such a good time producing great food for appreciative Texans," she told her literary agent, Elizabeth Ann Johnson. She miraculously turned out fancy dinners despite World War II rationing. Unable to get Wesson oil, she reportedly bought No. 1 refined mineral oil from the Humble Oil Company and used it for cooking purposes. "The people at the Houston Country Club were awfully healthy while I was there," she told Sweeney.

Joske's department store in Houston hired her away from the country club to manage its restaurant and catering, but the job wasn't a good fit. "Being fired from Joske's [for not bringing in enough money and not seeing eye to eye with the executives] was the best thing that ever happened to me," she said. She returned to Austin in the early fifties to reign over the Driskill Hotel's dining room and catering, introducing politicians and other dignitaries to food creatively prepared and properly served. Clarence "Captain" White, whom she trained to oversee the Driskill dining room, remembers, "When we served fresh asparagus [a truly exotic vegetable in those days], she always had us cut it on the bias, so it would look like green beans. The men would sometimes say, 'What kind of green beans are these? I like 'em!'" Recalls Lady Bird Johnson: "When Lyndon and Jesse Kellam had dinner parties at the Driskill, they always knew the evening would go well if Helen Corbitt was in charge." According to Bess Abell, the White House social secretary in the Johnson years, Helen Corbitt recipes were frequently used at the White House. Her signature flowerpot dessert was a natural for Mrs. Johnson's beautification luncheons. Years before anybody had heard of Martha Stewart, Corbitt layered tiny clay flowerpots with cake and ice cream, stuck a trimmed drinking straw in the middle, and topped off the pot with meringue. After the meringue was browned in the oven, she inserted a fresh flower in each straw. These desserts frequently pop up at Texas bridesmaids luncheons even today.

In 1955, after being courted for several years, Corbitt finally agreed to take over Neiman Marcus's food service. It is difficult to say who benefited more from the relationship. Neiman's flagship Dallas store was in its heyday. Texans had money and were spending it. Women still wore hats and gloves downtown, and the Zodiac Room, where men and women sipped Corbitt's tiny cups of chicken consommé while sleek models sporting the latest fashions circled their tables, was an oasis of sophistication and glamour. Corbitt had the flair, the taste, and the energy to produce food that was as visually enchanting as the store's windows on Main and Commerce. She was a cosmopolitan woman with a thorough knowledge of the best restaurants and food suppliers in the country. She was the first woman to win the Golden Plate Award, the highest honor in the food industry. She also garnered top honors from the gourmet society Confrérie de la Chaîne des Rotisseurs and served on the board of governors of the Culinary Institute of America. But most important, she understood Texans and delighted in getting them to eat foods that they professed to abhor, like lamb, anchovies, and yogurt. The assurance of good taste that Neiman Marcus's customers sought in the store's chic ready-to-wear could now be extended to their dining tables as well. "When Miss Corbitt put white grapes, heavy cream, and slivered toasted almonds in her chicken salad, it gave the rest of us confidence to experiment a bit," says one of her ardent followers.

The experiments didn't always work. Mary Bloom, who worked at Neiman's as a young woman, remembers asking Miss Corbitt to take a look at a dinner party menu she was planning for friends. "I'm trying to be creative the way you are," Mary said. "See, I'm going to peel the cantaloupe and stuff it with Roquefort cheese." Miss Corbitt paused and then, unleashing her famous Irish wit, said, "Mary, am I the first to tell you that you're pregnant?" She was.

The fabulous Neiman Marcus Foreign Fortnights, which the flagship store has recently resurrected, were launched in 1957. These were extravaganzas that took years to plan. Fortnights from France, Italy, Scandinavia, Great Britain, and Ireland brought to town not only the merchandise of those countries but their culture as well, in the form of concerts, art exhibits, film screenings, theater performances, and of course, food and wine. Corbitt was sent abroad to study the cuisine firsthand, and her adventures in foreign kitchens made great copy for her newspaper column, "Kitchen Klatter," which appeared in the *Houston Post* and the *Arkansas Gazette*. Sometimes European chefs were imported to her Zodiac kitchen. In her 1974 cookbook, *Helen Corbitt Cooks for Company*, she remembers a French chef and his assistants: "They asked for and received everything they wanted except the skin from a sheep's belly (I didn't know any sheep) and women (I . . . didn't know the right kind)." After they plied her kitchen staff with wine and brandy one day, she reclaimed her throne and declared that for future fortnights, she would research the recipes herself and do what she always did best, adapt the food to Texans' taste. She knew that we really wouldn't miss having our spinach puréed through a sheep's belly.

Stanley Marcus, in a foreword to a posthumous collection of Corbitt's recipes, wrote of her fourteen-year tenure at the helm of the Zodiac Room: "She was difficult, for she knew the difference between better and best, and she was never willing to settle for second best." He dubbed her his Wild Irish Genius and the Balenciaga of Food and kept her happy all those years by offering her daily compliments. "Too many chefs today regard themselves first as artists," Marcus says. "Corbitt created a beautiful plate, but she gave greater attention to how the food would taste." As a matter of fact, her meatloaf baked in an angel-food-cake tin really does taste better.

Corbitt had what these days we might call healthy self-esteem. She told Julia Sweeney about the time a produce clerk caught her picking out the freshest mushrooms in the back room at the Simon David specialty food store and said, "I'm sorry, but the manager doesn't allow people back here." She blithely responded, "Go tell the manager Helen Corbitt is here. I have pickin' privileges." Even Stanley Marcus recalls with amazement how quickly Helen could reduce a directive from the boss to a suggestion. In *Cooks for Company* she admitted that she sometimes forgot that she didn't own the Zodiac Room. Once, when the two sittings for a Fortnight dinner filled quickly, she decreed a third sitting, forgetting that it would entail keeping the entire store—with its lights, air conditioning, elevator operators, and security guards—open additional hours. She really caught it the next day, she wrote, but from then on there were three sittings. Corbitt's perfectionism exacted a price: Even though it was packed with people daily, the Zodiac Room never showed a profit. In his memoir *Minding the Store* Marcus wrote that, when he complained of heavy losses, she replied, "You didn't mention money when you employed me. You simply said that you wanted the best food in the country. I've given you that."

Soups in the Zodiac Room were always made from scratch, with one exception: the cream of tomato. In a 1972 interview with journalist Francis Raffetto, Corbitt admitted, "I used Campbell's, with coffee cream and butter to make it like velvet." New York playwright Moss Hart, having lunch one day in the late fifties with Marcus's brother Edward, ordered a second bowl and then asked for the recipe. To Marcus's chagrin, Corbitt refused. She later explained, "We couldn't tell Moss Hart he ate Campbell's soup at Neiman Marcus."

Helen Corbitt cooked for the smartly dressed country club set and for movie stars and socialites slimming at the Greenhouse Spa in Arlington, which she helped to create. She entertained royalty and the dignitaries of many foreign countries, but she also cooked for the secretaries and shopgirls and housewives who sometimes treated themselves to a pastry or a sandwich at the standup counter on the main floor. "Each bite of those little sandwiches was like a gift," one woman recalls. "They were generously spread, and there was always something surprising in a Helen Corbitt sandwich—a little pineapple in the tuna, a bit of chutney with the turkey—that made your tastebuds come to attention."

Even before she retired from Neiman Marcus in 1969, the indefatigable Corbitt was expanding her legacy, lecturing all over the country and writing cookbooks—her first, *Helen Corbitt's Cookbook* (1957), had more than 27 printings and sold more than 300,000 copies. Her cookbooks, now out of print, are a staple of every Texas cook's library. Worn-out copies, dog-eared and grease-splattered, are often rebound. Women who have cooked from her books all their lives light up with gratitude when her name is mentioned. "She taught me that I could entertain in a small apartment or in my kitchen without hired help," says a friend who used to have a catering business ("Just throw a clean white cup towel over the dirty dishes in the sink!" Corbitt suggested in one of her lectures).

Corbitt-trained cooks have their favorite recipes: the poppy-seed dressing for fruit salad; the pancake stack, ten to twelve very thin fourteen-inch pancakes, spread either with lemon-cream butter and hot blueberry sauce or with butter, maple syrup, and a little ham gravy, stacked, and sliced for serving like a pie; or perhaps the queen of desserts, caramel soufflé with English custard sauce.

Of the latter, wrote Corbitt in *Cooks for Company*, "You may halve the recipe, but why? Regardless of how few guests you have, it will all be eaten."

The generous party spirit, awash in butter, cream cheese, eggs, and mayonnaise, that pervades her first two cookbooks (the second, *Helen Corbitt's Potluck*, was published in 1962) inevitably gave way to the low-cholesterol, low-cal recipe collections, *Helen Corbitt Cooks for Looks* (1967) and *Helen Corbitt's Greenhouse Cookbook* (1979). Corbitt, like the rest of us, was fighting her own weight and cholesterol, and she refused to be limited to grapefruit and cottage cheese. Gone are the jaunty comments "Men will really love this" or "When you're feeling extravagant . . . ," but a number of good cooks swear by her simple roast chicken stuffed with grapes.

With missionary zeal, Corbitt shared her expertise. She taught cooking classes to benefit the Dallas Symphony, raising more than $150,000. She also taught a more intimate class of close friends and their daughters in the store, charging only for the food used in the demonstrations. The notes from those sessions are now being passed like heirlooms to a third generation. And she taught a rather exclusive cooking class for fourteen men—some doctors and businessmen, an oil man, a lawyer, a stockbroker, and a liquor-chain vice president—on Wednesday nights in her duplex on University. Corbitt, who never married, clearly enjoyed her male following, and her cookbooks are most often dedicated to them. She liked that men asked questions and wanted to know the "why" of certain procedures. "She also liked that she could give us hell without worrying that she'd hurt our feelings," recalls one of her male pupils, who still cooks her osso buco. She believed men were more adventurous in their food tastes and were held back by wives who just didn't want to learn to cook new things. Had she lived to see it, she would be especially saddened by women today who take the same pride in not cooking that women of a previous generation took in their inability to type or take shorthand. She was a hardworking professional who understood that to make a savory beef stew, a busy working woman might have to brown the meat one day and simmer it the next, but she believed there was pleasure to be found in cooking for people you loved. "The dining room is one of the last outposts of civilization," she wrote in *Cooks for Company.* "Let's keep it that way."

Helen Corbitt died of cancer in 1978. In the last year of her life, her good friend Father Don Fischer (now monsignor), then a young chaplain at the University of Dallas, took her the Eucharist daily. "It was a great gift to be able to bring spiritual food to such a lover of food," he says. "Even in her weakening condition, she always felt she should offer me something when I came to see her. I tried to beg off but finally said, 'Okay, but make it just something very simple.' She made me the best peanut-butter-and-jelly sandwich I've ever had. I know the bread was probably homemade. She spread it with butter, then a generous amount of peanut butter and marvelous preserves. I went away thinking that if that was what peanut butter and jelly was supposed to taste like, I had been a very deprived child."

In Texas, B.C., most of us were.

*December 1999*

# LADIES, FIRST

PATRICIA SHARPE

W hat's it like to be the state's entertainer in chief? Three former Texas first ladies and the current one dish about life in the mansion and share their favorite recipes.

AT NINE O'CLOCK IN THE MORNING on June 10, four of the six living first ladies of Texas—Anita Perry, Linda Gale White, Rita Clements, and Nellie Connally—assembled on the porch of the Governor's Mansion for brunch and a historic photograph. (Laura Bush and Jean Daniel were unable to attend.) There was no particular occasion for the picture, no anniversary or holiday. We asked the women if they would let us photograph them simply because we thought it was high time they were recognized for doing a job that too often goes unremarked: that of entertainer in chief.

As sunlight fell across the building's tall white columns, I watched as the four of them smiled for the camera, obligingly moved a step to the right and then to the left, stood up, sat down, and smiled some more. During breaks, the three former first ladies strolled about the building and gardens to see what had changed since they left and to say hello to employees they had known. It was like a reunion of members of the state's most exclusive club.

Far more than governors do, first ladies practice pragmatic politics. They understand that while they are expected to support worthy charities and deliver speeches, their role as hostess is equally significant. They learn the political value of a well-set table laden with prime rib, mashed potatoes, grilled asparagus, and chocolate mousse. Moreover, they understand the subtle (and not-so-subtle) power of good dining to make guests feel contented, magnanimous, and beholden. When I asked the first ladies if they would let us publish a recipe from their time at the mansion, they immediately agreed.

Later, when I called to ask a few questions about their culinary interests and what it was like to live in the historic home, it felt more like talking to friends than doing interviews (the fact that I wasn't trying to dig up dirt on the governor or the kids didn't hurt). Anita Perry told me that she loves to read cookbooks (she owns about 75) and that since she was a child, her favorite dish has been buttered grits; Governor Rick Perry's favorite dishes are his wife's fried chicken and buttermilk pie. During Laura Bush's tenure as first lady, the mansion kitchen turned out an array of dishes with a Texas and Southwestern orientation. One—a spicy snack called Sarah's Chex Mix, after mansion chef Sarah Bishop Ninaud— even made national headlines when the White House had to call Ninaud to get the recipe just right. Linda Gale White recalled that one day in 1983, the cook fixed a dessert so unpalatable that the White children sneaked out the back door and dumped their servings into the flower bed. When Rita Clements moved into the then-123-year-old structure, in 1979, it was so decrepit and the kitchen so cramped that food for large events had to be temporarily stored in the garage; she and Governor Bill Clements initiated a major renovation project. Nellie Connally, who told one funny story after another, remembered that when her family moved into the mansion, in 1963, the china cabinet had exactly two serving pieces. "One was a bowl—a flower bowl, actually," she said, "and the other was a platter that looked like it had come in a box of laundry soap." Jean Daniel, a descendant of former Texas governor Sam Houston, always had fresh-baked sugar cookies on hand for her four children when she was first lady, from 1957 to 1963.

Talking to the first ladies, however briefly, whetted my appetite for more details, especially about some of their predecessors. So I turned to Austinite Carl McQueary, a member of the Texas Historical Commission and the author of a forthcoming cookbook and culinary history of the mansion that will be published by Texas A&M University Press next year. I had seen part of the manuscript and was intrigued. "So, Carl," I asked, "what's the most unusual dish ever prepared at the Governor's Mansion?" He replied, "Well, they had bear once," then added, "Why don't I just send you a copy of the whole book?" In due course an e-mail arrived with a monster attachment: 450 pages. In the time it took to print it, I could have roasted a buffalo like the one Governor W. Lee "Pappy" O'Daniel served at his inaugural party in 1941.

Although I was vastly disappointed that the book did not contain a recipe for buffalo (or bear, for that matter), I still found it a fascinating window onto Texas history. I discovered that the Governor's Mansion has been no rarefied repository of haute cuisine. At any given period, the food served there reflected what ordinary people were eating. Yes, the mansion cooks prepared fancy fare for official dinners, but even those dishes were never too far removed from the mainstream. The other interesting thing is how the mainstream has changed over the years. A typical pot of coffee in Governor Sam Houston's day (the mid-nineteenth century), for example, would take the bristles off a hog. Brewing the stuff entailed boiling a cup of freshly ground coffee beans and a crushed eggshell in six cups of water for three minutes; the liquid was then strained into cups containing beaten egg whites, cream, and lots of sugar. Breakfast was a much bigger deal in the past than it is today. During the administration of Governor James S. Hogg (1891–1895), the kitchen staff regularly cooked fried eggs, home-cured ham, grits with redeye gravy, a choice of butter biscuits or cornmeal hotcakes with ribbon cane syrup, and oatmeal with cream or clabber (similar to yogurt). No wonder the estimable governor weighed nearly three hundred pounds.

But the flip side of these culinary oddities is an equal number of recipes that have an enduring appeal. Homey comfort foods haven't changed at all—Orlene Sayers' coconut cake, dating from around 1900, would be at home on any dinner table today, as would Miriam "Ma" Ferguson's chili, served during the twenties, and Margaret Lea Houston's fried green tomatoes. The most common recipes are for corn pone, corn cakes, and their fancier descendant, cornbread; Jell-O desserts (the stuff was being marketed as early as 1900); and cakes, cookies, and biscuits. Indeed, if any one food embodies the heart and soul of Texas cuisine, as served in the Governor's Mansion over the years, it would have to be biscuits. The aforementioned Governor O'Daniel was elected at least in part because of a song that he wrote, "Please Pass the Biscuits, Pappy." (He also inspired the character of Mississippi governor Menelaus "Pappy" O'Daniel in the 2000 hit movie *O Brother, Where Art Thou?*)

So it's fitting that for this story, Nellie Connally supplied a recipe for biscuits. She told me that they were first made by a mansion cook named Annie Menzel and that they are best when served with lots of butter and honey. "I could eat a whole plateful about now," she said. Me too.

## GRILLED SHRIMP–PASTA SALAD

*ANITA PERRY*

### Pasta with Vinaigrette

½ cup olive oil
2 tablespoons red wine vinegar
2 tablespoons lemon juice
1 tablespoon Dijon mustard
2 cloves garlic, minced
1 tablespoon finely chopped assorted herbs (your choice of
    fresh basil, oregano, tarragon, rosemary, etc.)
kosher salt and freshly ground pepper to taste
8 ounces uncooked rotelle (spiral pasta)

To make vinaigrette, whisk all ingredients except the pasta in a bowl and set aside. Cook pasta according to package directions, drain, and toss with vinaigrette while still warm. Set aside. Do not prepare more than about 30 minutes in advance.

### Marinade for Shrimp

1 cup olive oil
4 cloves garlic, minced
2 tablespoons minced fresh rosemary

(or 1 tablespoon dried)
1 teaspoon kosher salt

Combine ingredients in a bowl and set aside.

### Shrimp and Vegetables

2 pounds raw shrimp
2 carrots, peeled
1 yellow squash, halved lengthwise
1 zucchini, halved lengthwise
1 red bell pepper, halved lengthwise
1 yellow bell pepper, halved lengthwise
1 yellow onion, quartered
olive oil, for brushing on vegetables
salt and pepper to taste
2 tablespoons coarsely chopped flat-leaf parsley

Heat charcoal grill. Peel and devein shrimp, place in marinade, and set aside. Brush vegetables with olive oil and arrange on grill about 6 inches from heat. Grill until tender, then cut into bite-size pieces. Arrange shrimp on skewers and grill, turning once, until opaque and cooked through, about 4 minutes (do not overcook). Toss vegetables and shrimp with pasta. Add salt and pepper. Just before serving, stir in chopped parsley. Serves 6.

## TOMATO ASPIC

### RITA CLEMENTS

2 ½ tablespoons unflavored gelatin
1 quart tomato juice (4 cups)
1 small can spicy tomato juice, such as V-8 or Bloody Mary
    mix
1 ½ teaspoons salt
¼ teaspoon finely ground black pepper
6 whole cloves
2 bay leaves
1 tablespoon sugar

1 ½ teaspoons powdered mustard

dash Worcestershire sauce

1 medium onion, puréed in a food processor or grated by
hand, including juice

1 additional medium onion, finely chopped (optional, if you
especially like onion)

1 cup finely chopped celery

1 ½2 cup finely chopped green bell pepper

Note: You will need 8 individual molds.

In a large bowl, dissolve gelatin in ¼ cup water (takes about 5
minutes). Meanwhile, place next 9 ingredients in a saucepan over
high heat and bring to a simmer. Reduce heat and continue simmering for 15 minutes. Strain, then pour over the dissolved gelatin
and stir. Let cool to about room temperature, then stir in onion,
celery, and bell pepper.

Pour into molds and refrigerate until gelatin sets, about
2 hours. To unmold, invert onto a platter and cover with a hot,
damp towel or cloth until loosened. Serves 8.

### SOUTHWESTERN POTATO SALAD

*LAURA BUSH*

12 medium red potatoes, with or without skins

2 to 3 pickled jalapeños, chopped (seeded if desired)

¼ to ½ cup chopped Kalamata olives

3 to 4 teaspoons whole-grain mustard

¾ cup mayonnaise, or to taste

2 teaspoons chopped fresh cilantro

2 teaspoons chopped fresh oregano

2 large eggs, hard-cooked and diced

salt and pepper to taste

Boil potatoes in salted water until cooked, about 20 minutes.
Rinse in cool water. When cool enough to handle, cut potatoes
into bite-size cubes. While still warm, toss with remaining ingredients. Adjust seasonings. Chill for at least 2 hours before serving.
Serves 6.

## ORANGE-ZEST BISCUITS

*NELLIE CONNALLY*

2 cups flour
4 tablespoons sugar
½ teaspoon salt
2 ½ teaspoons baking powder
5 tablespoons vegetable shortening
zest of 1 orange, grated or finely chopped
½ cup milk
½ cup orange juice

Preheat oven to 425 degrees. Sift dry ingredients together. Cut in shortening and then stir in orange zest. Combine milk and orange juice, add to flour mixture, and stir with a fork until dough is fairly free from sides of bowl, no more than half a minute. Pat dough out ¾ inch thick on a lightly floured surface and cut with a 2-inch biscuit cutter. Bake until golden brown, about 15 minutes. Makes about 16.

## STRAWBERRY—CREAM CHEESE STARS

*LINDA GALE WHITE*

8 ounces cream cheese, softened
¼ cup confectioners' sugar
⅛ teaspoon cinnamon
1 tablespoon lemon juice
1 quart fresh strawberries

Using an electric mixer, combine first 4 ingredients in a mixing bowl and beat until smooth; cover and refrigerate. Clean and hull strawberries (holes should be about ½ inch in diameter). Place on a paper towel, open side down, and dry thoroughly. With a small knife, cut an X in each strawberry, starting at the pointed end and continuing about ¾ of the way through. Gently open each berry, and using a pastry bag with a large star tip, pipe cream-cheese filling into its cavity. (If this is too much trouble, you can omit cutting the X and just fill the hollow of each berry with cream-cheese mixture.) They may be served in paper petit-four cups. Makes about 3 dozen.

## FAVORITE COOKIES

### JEAN DANIEL

    1 cup unsalted butter, softened
    1 cup sugar
    1 cup brown sugar
    2 eggs, lightly beaten
    1 teaspoon baking soda
    1 teaspoon salt
    1 teaspoon vanilla extract
    2 cups pecan pieces
    4 cups flour

Using an electric mixer, beat butter with sugar and brown sugar until creamy. Beat in eggs, baking soda, salt, and vanilla. Stir in pecans. Stir in flour, in 3 or 4 batches.

Tear off 6 pieces of waxed paper or plastic wrap, each about 18 inches long. Divide dough into 6 equal portions and shape each into a log about 6 inches long. Wrap each portion of dough in the waxed paper or plastic wrap and refrigerate until firm, at least 1 hour.

Preheat oven to 325 degrees. Cut rolls into ¼-inch-thick slices and bake on an ungreased cookie sheet until golden brown, 12 to 15 minutes. Cool on a rack. Makes 2 dozen.

Recipes adapted from *Cooking at the Governor's Mansion* by Carl R. McQueary, published by Texas A&M University Press in 2003.

*August 2002*

# HOW TO OPEN A RESTAURANT

PATRICIA SHARPE

$S$ome assembly required. Silverware not included.

I WAS SITTING AT MY DESK earlier this year wondering if anyone would notice if I left for lunch at ten-thirty when the phone rang. Cruelly torn from my reverie of cheese enchiladas, I picked up the receiver. On the line were Lisa and Emmett Fox, Austin chefs and restaurateurs, who had an offer that no food critic in her right mind could refuse: "We're opening a new restaurant," they said. "Wanna watch?" I asked them to hold for a minute while I cleared my calendar. And that is how I got to be—I was about to say "a fly on the wall," but that seems an unfortunate metaphor—an embedded reporter chronicling the highs and lows of the eight-month gestation of Fino Restaurant, Patio, and Bar.

For three decades I've been looking on as fledgling dining establishments struggle to open—often behind schedule and hopelessly muddled—so I was prepared for Murphy's Law to operate with a vengeance. But if anybody could survive the ordeal relatively unscathed, I thought, it was the Foxes, for the compelling reason that they had already opened one successful restaurant. At their five-year-old neighborhood place, Asti Trattoria, Emmett acts as paterfamilias to his staff and customers and Lisa takes care of business. A big bear of a man, Emmett graduated from the Culinary Institute of America, in Hyde Park, New York; Lisa, who is shyer than you would expect for someone so pretty, studied art at the University of Massachusetts in Amherst. But their experience isn't limited to Asti. Emmett worked at the chic Cafe Annie, in Houston, and was executive chef for a restaurant group in Austin that included the Granite Cafe. Lisa, whose specialty is pastry, was in demand for her lavish desserts at several tony places around town. Now that Asti was running smoothly, they couldn't resist the lure of, well, having a second child.

By the time of our first meeting, in February, the two had already decided that their new baby would be Mediterranean. Casual but stylish, its menu would emphasize small plates meant for sharing. Wines would be important, especially interesting, affordable European ones. They even had a name picked out: Fino. The word refers to a type of dry Spanish sherry and also means "fine" in both Spanish and Italian—surely a good omen. And they had a location, which by coincidence was Emmett's old stomping grounds, the now-defunct Granite Cafe. True, the interior needed an extreme makeover—it had last looked cool when Ronald Reagan was president—but otherwise, it was perfect: space for around a hundred, plenty of parking, and, sexiest of all, a covered patio. Another bonus: The landlord, Jim Holden, owner of the Live Oak Group real estate development company, was so tickled to have a major tenant back in the vacant space that he had agreed to pay for major improvements.

As for the rest of the money to support this addition to their family? After circulating a 32-page business proposal before Christmas, complete with a mouthwatering sample menu (lamb chops with couscous and feta, pistachio baklava with honey ice cream), the Foxes had ended up with eight investors: four of the five who had funded Asti, Lisa's two brothers, her doctor, and her doctor's mother. It took two months to raise $400,000, in shares of $50,000 and $25,000. Having acquired the money, they immediately started depleting it by hiring a project designer: Michael Hsu, a partner with the prestigious Dick Clark Architecture. Low key, almost Zen-like, Michael, out of all the candidates they interviewed, had the most practical knowledge about restaurants. "He told us stuff like the restrooms and stove hood not being up to code," Emmett said. And in going with Dick Clark's firm, they got a package deal: Equally unflappable interior designer Kasey McCarty was assigned to the project. They were ready to go.

## EARLY FEBRUARY

One cold winter afternoon, I sit down with the Foxes at Asti to play catch-up. The staff is preparing dinner, and I can see Emmett's eyes following everything in the open kitchen. One of the big things I want to know is this: Did you or Michael come up with Fino's look? "We talked in broad strokes," says Lisa. "It was a feeling, more than details." They envisioned the space as divided into two sections, a quieter dining side and a lively lounge side. But their specific mandates were few: Incorporate wood and the color orange into the plans, and don't do anything too trendy. Wood and orange? I ask, baffled. They lend a warm, Mediterranean feel, Lisa says. And why nothing too modern? So the look won't get dated. Michael's solution has three key elements: a sleek, blond paneled bar in the middle of the room, an intricate wood screen behind the bar, and a floor-to-ceiling "wine wall" with built-in wood racks. As for orange, he's leaving that up to Kasey. The three of us talk for a good hour, but when Emmett starts to jump up every two minutes, I figure I've worn out my welcome. On my way out the door, I call out one last question: "When are you opening?" "Mid-MAY," they shout back, "if we're lucky."

FEBRUARY 23: It's my first meeting with the Fino crew, and we're all crowded around the groovy conference table at Dick Clark's office.

The idea is to meet here every Tuesday at eleven to hash out details until the plans are final; once construction starts, we'll meet at Fino. Lisa and Emmett I know, of course, and I feel like I've already met Michael and Kasey. Dick Clark is sitting in today (he likes to kid around and serves as a nice leavening agent); also on hand is Carey Dodson, a designer who's assisting Michael. Here from Asti is Brian Stubbs, who with his mop of sandy hair resembles a tall, blond Beatle. He's slated to become Fino's manager. And representing the building end is Beth Selbe Lasita, the owner of Pinnacle Construction. Frankly, I've never met a contractor like Beth, who wears ruffly skirts and mules but can talk hood chases and fire-rated wraps with the best of them. Maybe it's just because I'm taking notes and everybody is on their best behavior, but the inevitable disagreements are being handled with impressive diplomacy. If I expected shouting and pouting, it hasn't happened yet.

Everybody's got their calendars and PDAs out, and big sheaves of architectural drawings are unrolled. Today's goal is to finalize the building plans so Beth can advertise for bids; Kasey needs to get started too, selecting furniture and fabrics. But in fact, the discussion is all over the map, and soon I wish I had a *Building for Dummies* to explain all the technical terms and acronyms: HVAC, elevations, TAS, Lumacite, lap-and-gap. There's a mountain of minutiae to be dealt with, like how tall to make the banquettes ("Just high enough so you can see waiters' heads going back and forth, like a puppet show," offers Dick) and how many restroom stalls the city codes require. It's a long meeting, and after a while, Dick disappears and returns with cappuccinos for everybody. When we finish, with plans still not final, Emmett and Michael head off to a showroom to look at flooring. Beth agrees to come back in three weeks with estimates. The meetings may be just once a week, but the work never stops.

EARLY MARCH

Speaking of work, one of the main hurdles in opening a restaurant is getting a liquor license. Booze doesn't just keep the customers happy, it helps pay the bills, and the Foxes expect a third of Fino's sales to be beer, wine, and cocktails. So it's crucial to be nicey-nice to the lovely people at the Texas Alcoholic Beverage Commission. To handle the paperwork, the Foxes have hired a professional facilitator, Carole Terry-Gonynor. In a calm voice that leads me to believe she might have once been a horse whisperer, Carole explains that the worst part isn't paying the license fee ($1,250 in Fino's case). The headache is the background checks. Once again, I'm mystified. Background checks? Carole says that restaurants and bars have so routinely been used to launder money by or-

ganized crime, drug moguls, and crooked businessmen that the
TABC is now required to compile records on liquor license applicants and their financial backers. Lisa's distressed over having
to ask her investors nosy questions, but Carole assures her, ever so
soothingly, that Fino will have a license by mid-May at the latest.
Famous last words.

MARCH 8: We're huddled around the conference table,
knee to knee, and Michael and Emmett are jabbing at a spot on
the plans and looking exasperated. Emmett would dearly love to
move a bulky, three-compartment sink, but the health regs say it
has to be in a certain place, never mind the inconvenience. Grinning, Dick sums up everybody's frustration: "Bureaucracy makes
the job so much more fun." Other problems are trotted out, some
solved, most not. Several times, the subject of cost comes up. I've
noticed—we've all noticed—that the laundry list of stuff they
hope Jim the landlord will pay for is growing . . . and growing . . .
and growing: the air conditioning, maybe the vent hood, the
kitchen floor, the drains. After a bit, Lisa says, "I'll call him today to let him know what's going on." Dick adds, "We'll get him
pumped." They hope.

MARCH 15: Kasey walks in and dumps an armload of up-
holstery books, wood samples, and pieces of fabric on the conference table. You can tell before she arranges them that these
combinations are way cool. The geometric patterns are retro but
not stodgy. The colors—apple green, espresso, taupe, and, *yes*, a
reddish orange—pop. Lisa breathes in sharply and says, "Yeah!"
Emmett's a little dubious. "If you're sure about those patterns
working together," he says, winking at Lisa, "I better be." Next,
Kasey opens a catalog and turns to a picture of a wild light fixture
made out of Campari bottles. Everybody loves it. The price is a
lot—$445. But, what the hell, they pencil two of them into the
decor budget.

MARCH 18: You know when you get news so terrible that
you can't even react, you just stare? Beth's bid is on the table,
and they're all looking at the figures in utter disbelief. The total
is a staggering $130,000 over budget. Most of it isn't even for the
glamour stuff; it's for plumbing, air conditioning, and electrical

work. For once, Dick's office is a glum place. Over the next hour the group fine-tooth-combs the budget, paring off a few thousand dollars here and there but nothing major. The more they talk, the more it seems as if the only hope is for the cavalry—i.e., Jim—to come riding in and save the day. "Can some of the stove hood be split off to his column?" Lisa wonders. "What about the patio things, like heaters and gas lines?" somebody else says. It's a lot to expect, and they know it. Finally there is nothing else to do but wait till Beth can revise the specifications and get new bids, re-jigger the columns, and hope that Jim is in a generous mood.

MARCH 20: In the meantime, it's time for something fun: the menu. We're out at the Foxes' airy "Texan-Tuscan" house tonight for one of several recipe-testing sessions. Emmett and Lisa are cooking, and so is Tristan White, the Asti day chef who's moving over to head up Fino's kitchen. Quiet, with a sly little smile and a stupendous tattoo of a samurai and a fish on one arm, Tristan graduated from culinary school in his native Australia. Also here are Brian, Fino's manager, and Boris Krouse, the courtly, wry wine steward from Asti, who will play the same role at Fino. To say that Boris is interested in wine is like saying that cats are mildly aroused by catnip.

Tristan is doing French onion soup. Emmett is roasting a Moroccan-spiced shoulder of lamb and making a version of some potatoes with garlic aioli that he and Lisa once had in Barcelona. "They were fantastic," he tells me. Also planned are a seafood paella and a Spanish *crema catalana*, a flanlike dessert. I get underfoot and annoy them with questions, like, Where *do* you get ideas for a brand-new menu? Turns out that the process is eminently simple: They read cookbooks, dozens of them. "We all look at them whenever we have a spare minute," says Emmett. And they travel. They've gone to a couple of Mediterranean-style restaurants in Houston (Ibiza and Rioja) and nearly a score of all types in San Francisco. Their visit to the California city also gave them the idea of doing one of the first community tables in Austin, which will be a great focal point for the dining room.

But tonight, they're seeing if the dishes that sound so good actually taste good. An hour passes, and gradually the house fills with fantastic smells. Another hour crawls by, and just when several of us are preparing to storm the kitchen with pitchforks, the food is ready. We eat, and then they spend half an hour in a roundtable discussion systematically picking apart each and every dish. And I thought restaurant critics were mean.

MARCH 21: Ah, another change of scenery. Emmett, Lisa, and Brian are at the local office of the international design firm Pentagram, sitting around *its* groovy conference table, while graphic designer Lowell Williams tosses out trial menu covers like cards from a deck. With his round black glasses, à la the late architect Philip Johnson, Lowell cuts quite the eccentric figure. The first of his three samples has stripes, a bit like the Italian flag; the second shows a picture of a cork with "FINO" printed on it. The third takes each letter of "Fino" and enlarges it to fill an entire page, so that some menu covers have a single large *F*, others a large *I*, and so on. It's a hip, clean look. Lisa approves. As for signs, Lowell wants to stencil "FINO Restaurant Patio Bar" directly on the wall of the building, like a stock-market ticker. "We can make it great big, like a frieze," he says. "It will also cost thousands of dollars less." Lisa says, "Thousands less? I *love* it."

MARCH 22: The tension is as thick as the foam on one of Dick's cappuccinos. Jim is here to look at the budget. Everyone is sitting at the conference table with tight little smiles on their faces. When Jim asks, "Have you all seen the costs?" Brian jokes, "Yeah, Emmett didn't have any gray in his hair a week ago." Michael begins the meeting by explaining the overall design; then Kasey describes the decor. They're all watching Jim like cats at a mouse hole. He smiles and says, "Neat." Then Beth takes a breath and says, "I always get the fun part," and hands around a spreadsheet. The total in the landlord's column has got to be tens of thousands of dollars more than he expected. Beth finishes her spiel, and at first it seems like things are all right. Jim smiles again and says, "I love the design, and I am really excited about it all." Then his smile fades. "However," he goes on, "these numbers *far* exceed the scope of the agreement and discussions I've had with Emmett and Lisa. We are way, way, way, *way, way, way* apart, and under no scenario am I prepared to put in that amount without contemplating it first." Dead silence. Then he turns to Emmett and Lisa and says, "The three of us need to sit down and discuss this—alone."

Emmett asks, "Now?" Jim says, "Yes." They get up and leave. Dick turns to me with a grin: "I think your backstage pass just got revoked." No kidding.

I don't get a call from Lisa till late afternoon. Has Jim pulled out? Is this the end? Finally the phone rings. Whew! Good news: He's still on board and they have another meeting planned. Lisa sounds chastened but philosophical. "You know, we hadn't wanted to bother him with too much detail along the way," she says, "but in hindsight, maybe we should have—except we didn't know ourselves until last Friday." Bottom line, she and Emmett have crunched some numbers and they think the job is going to cost more like $500,000 than $400,000. And that means two things: slashing the budget and raising more money. "But we'll figure it out," she says softly. "We can still have a fantastic restaurant."

APRIL 11: Major progress. Lisa calls to say that, after several agonizing meetings, they've shaved $55,000 off the project. They axed some of the patio shutters and the outdoor heat lamps and, sadly, eliminated the Campari light fixtures. To save more, Michael and Carey have redesigned the wine wall and the entrance. "The design is now as tight as it can be," Lisa tells me. The other good—actually, fantastic—news is that Jim has agreed to kick in a considerable additional amount for permanent improvements. On top of that, they've raised more money—two new investors at $25,000 each—and they've gotten a $100,000 line of credit at their bank to use if they need to. In short, they've saved the restaurant, but now there's another $50,000—maybe $150,000—to pay back. The actual date for construction to be done has now been set: JUNE 22. Fino is under the gun to succeed—fast.

APRIL 16: Road trip! Emmett and Tristan and I are in Houston at Joe Presswood's auction center so they can buy gently used equipment for Fino's kitchen. The plan all along has been to purchase some pieces new (refrigerators, for instance) and the rest old. Prowling around the huge, fluorescent-lit metal warehouse looking at stuff, we marvel at the endless rows of stoves, refrigerators, bar sinks, proofing ovens, stockpots big enough to cook a hippo, and one strange contraption that looks like R2-D2. The auction takes two days, but by the end, Emmett has a truckload of equipment to take home. More will be bought later.

MAY 10: Construction is under way, and our weekly meetings have moved to the Fino site. A month ago, it looked like something out of *Blade Runner*, with debris everywhere and a fine gray dust hanging in the air. Now walls are starting to take shape. When I arrive today, though, tape measures are out, a bad sign. Emmett is standing in the open corridor that will run between the kitchen, dining room, and bar, and he's pretty wound up. "The space is too tight," he's saying. "It won't work if a waiter has a tray of food and somebody else is picking up drinks." It turns out that the original, eighteen-year-old blueprints—on which the entire remodel is based—are seven inches short in one dimension. In his usual quiet mode, Michael turns to Mark Bridle, the job supervisor, and asks, "Can you move a wall?" Mark smiles weakly.

MAY 17: Lisa's fit to be tied. She expected to have a liquor license by now, but instead the TABC has kicked their application back for more investor information. "I just want to yell!" she says. The conversation turns to soft-drink suppliers. Brian's having a hard time with Coke. "They're prima donnas," he says. Somebody else says, "Oh, they're just jerks." Kasey says, "Yeah, soda jerks," and everybody cracks up. Lisa announces she's going shopping for bargain bathroom fixtures.

MAY 23: Fino's liquor license may have been sucked into the TABC twilight zone, but the restaurant eventually *will* need a wine list, and that calls for—wine tastings. Boris has been doing them systematically for weeks. His goal is to create a list of eighty wines evenly divided between white and red, ranging from $20 to $75. Around three o'clock he strolls into Fino with five wineglasses laced between his fingers, followed by Tristan with two Asti pizzas. We are meeting with Dana Harkrider, a rep from Ambiente wine distributors, to taste Spanish and Italian wines. While she sets up, Boris gets out some notepaper. In thirty minutes we've sampled five wines, some nice, others so-so. The last is a D'Anguera Finca L'Argata 2002, a Syrah-Cabernet blend from Spain. Boris inhales deeply. Glancing over his shoulder, I can see him writing "Violets plus plums . . . a beautiful nose." He takes a sip and scribbles some more: "Brooding yet lush." Have we been dropped into a scene from *Sideways?* Boris grins. "Like Marlene Dietrich's eyes," he jokes. He wants this wine bad, and Dana knows it. They wheel and deal, but tragically, Marlene Dietrich does not make it onto the wine list.

JUNE 7: Uh-oh. Somewhere along the way, numerous small construction delays have added up; the finish date is now JUNE 27. Meanwhile, it's breezy up here on Fino's patio, waiting for job applicants to show up. Ads have been running for the 36 positions that are available—13 in the kitchen, plus 23 servers, hosts, and bartenders. The mostly twentysomething interviewees are a mixed bag—some clean-cut, others who look as if they just rolled out of bed. Emmett says, "It's amazing to me that eighty percent of them didn't bring pens or pencils!" Boris and Brian are hiring the waiters, asking questions such as "Do you read cookbooks or cooking magazines?" and "Have you been criticized for anything?" After listening for a while, I can predict whom they will hire—those with experience and a smile and who don't seem terminally neurotic. But I'm surprised at whom Emmett and Tristan approve of. Initially, I'd assumed they would favor innovative cooks with strong ideas. Turns out that's the kiss of death. Yes, they insist on excellent skills, but they're rejecting anyone who wants to do things his way. Their attitude: Fino is *our* vision, dude; if you want to be creative, go raise half a million dollars and open your own damn restaurant.

JUNE 21: Amazing. The walls were painted two weeks ago, and furniture in Kasey's edgy colors has started to arrive. It really does look like a restaurant; even the long, tall community table is in place. Emmett, however, is steamed over something else. "C'mere," he says to me. A plumber has installed water pipes precisely where the custom-built walk-in cooler is supposed to go. Worse, the walk-in is missing in action: The man who was supposed to have ordered it has stopped returning Emmett's calls. This is major: If the walk-in doesn't come, construction can't be finished, the final health inspection won't happen, and the restaurant can't open. If the restaurant isn't open, there's no money to pay salaries, rent, and overhead except for the line of credit at the bank.

JUNE 27: The bad news is that construction was supposed to wrap today—and doesn't. The good news is that the errant cooler has been ordered and will arrive JULY 1, supposedly. But, hey, the deep-orange carpet and the blond-wood bar are in and looking good. Outside, two guys in a cherry picker are painting the words "FINO Restaurant Patio Bar" on the wall. Downstairs, Brian is running a three-day orientation session for the new hires, going over the sixteen-page employee's manual that he has written. (Under the section on appearance are the following Austin-centric rules: "No facial piercing," "No gum chewing," "No dark glasses.") Part of the orientation is a fifty-item wine quiz, courtesy of Boris. (Sample questions: "From what grape varietal is Sancerre made?" "Name five German viticultural regions." "Define 'dosage.'") *Merde!* Who but a sommelier could pass this monster?

JUNE 28: Lisa is freaking out. The liquor license *still* hasn't been approved. If they don't have it by opening night, they can kiss a third of their sales good-bye until it arrives. Downstairs, Brian is trying to bolster the morale of the new staff after just about everybody failed Boris's exam. Emmett and Lisa's dog, Lottie, ambles around the meeting room nuzzling everyone—cold comfort if you didn't know a noble grape from a bunghole.

JULY 1: I can hardly believe we've come so far: Tristan is actually ordering food and supplies—chickpeas, pistachio nuts, feta cheese, sea salt, truffle oil, figs, arborio rice, four kinds of paprika, white anchovies, pea shoots, and fresh mozzarella, not to mention trash bags, scrubbies, and cleaning rags. Of course, nothing can be delivered until the walk-in arrives. It's like being trapped in *Waiting for Godot*.

JULY 5: Hallelujah! The walk-in came three days ago and is now installed. Fino will go live next Monday night, six days from now. In the meantime, there are dozens of nitpicky things to correct. For one thing, the seats on the lounge chairs have to be exchanged because they're way too small. Somebody jokes, "I'd need a chair for each cheek." There's one more city inspection left, scheduled for Thursday. Tristan is bouncing up and down on his toes. "Once it's done," he says, "it's ready steady spaghetti."

JULY 8: Break out the champagne. "The TABC approved us!" Lisa announces, all smiles. More good news: The final city inspection happened yesterday morning. But there's still so much to do that opening night has now been postponed from Monday to Tuesday. Meanwhile, the aroma of baking pita bread wafts from the kitchen. In the dining room Michael, Kasey, Emmett, and Lisa are doing the final walk-through with the contractor's reps. Half-way through, somebody notices that—how can this be?—Tristan's name is written on the community table. Oh, *no!* The day before, he signed a carbon-paper form on the table, and the ink has penetrated its shiny surface. They try scrubbing it with water, saliva, window cleaner, lacquer thinner, bleach, paint remover, and a scary-sounding solvent named High-Flash Naphtha-150. Nothing works. At least Tristan's handwriting is small.

JULY 9: The young cooks who got the coveted jobs a month ago are learning all the new recipes, finding their way around the kitchen, and looking shell-shocked. Tristan is running the show now, and Emmett is trying to keep his mouth shut, although it's pretty hard when you're used to being the daddy. At three o'clock, the service staff is coming in for a mass tasting, and the kitchen staff is rushing to prepare every single dish on the menu. It's a madhouse, but there's really no choice. Food and liquor have been bought, and the meter is running. If they don't get this place open, they're screwed.

JULY 11: Fino's "soft opening," a complimentary feed for the investors and some 75 other invited guests, happens tonight. With candles flickering on the tables and a huge vase of flowers on the hostess stand, the restaurant looks stunning. The servers are wearing their new black T-shirts with "FINO" across the front, and you can see them nervously smiling and straining to remember what Brian has taught them: Put the menus down at a 45-degree angle across the place settings; don't drip ice water on the guests when you fill their glasses. My three friends and I are having a fine time and enjoying the food (which, by the way, is excellent), except for the fact that, well, to tell you the truth, it's starting to feel a little warm in here. Is the air conditioner on? By eight-thirty the temperature must be 95 degrees, and we're all sweating like John Goodman. At about nine-thirty the AC finally cranks up again—just before a tremendous *CRASH* resounds from the kitchen. A huge shelf of plates has pulled loose from the wall and smashed into a million pieces. Murphy's Law is kicking in right on schedule.

JULY 12: The big night: The restaurant welcomes its first patrons. Thank God the air conditioning has been fixed. When I arrive, Brian opens the door with a flourish and says, "Welcome to Fino!" In the kitchen, Tristan is cleaning salmon filets. Lisa is in the dining room hugging friends, looking dazed and happy. Emmett is alternately chatting with customers and expediting orders at the pass-through, yelling, "Trout—let's go!" Outside, the neighborhood folks who have been watching the construction for week after week are wandering in to check it all out. Boris says, "I'll bet by the end of the evening we have twenty-five paying customers." I'll bet he's right. For some reason, I stick around far longer than I need to, talking to Lisa, drinking sherry, finally closing my reporter's notebook altogether. The truth is, I'm having a little attack of postpartum depression. I don't want it to be over. When I finally walk out the door at nine o'clock, two more parties are coming in, and I hear Emmett shouting, "Hey, Tristan! It's a two-top and a six-top." Fino is open for business.

*September 2005*

# WE REMEMBER
# NINFA LAURENZO

 PATRICIA SHARPE

*S*he gave her name to a restaurant that revolutionized Mexican cooking, but she gave much more to the city of Houston.

WHEN HOUSTON RESTAURATEUR NINFA LAURENZO died in Houston in June at the age of 77, Texans who didn't even know her were surprised and saddened. Her face—the eyes crinkled into a smile of near-geothermal warmth—had become such an icon that the founder and owner of Ninfa's restaurants easily ranked among the five most recognized women in Houston. Of course, Ninfa's family and friends knew the seriousness of her two-year battle against breast cancer, but the thousands of others who were taken unawares felt as if they had lost a neighbor.

Ninfa's life was—no disrespect intended—a soap opera of epic proportions. She had been widowed at the age of 45 in 1969, when her husband, Domenic Laurenzo, died, leaving her to run their struggling tortilla and pizza-dough factory. Four years later, having mortgaged her house and having scraped together pots and pans from her own kitchen, she and the four eldest of her five children opened a ten-table restaurant in the front of the factory on Navigation Boulevard. The fledgling enterprise burned down two weeks later, but was quickly rebuilt. Within months, her little restaurant achieved enormous local popularity, and by the early nineties it had burgeoned to a chain of 35 units.

From the first day, Ninfa's was something different on the local scene. "Their food was like food from Mexico," says Fredericka Hunter, the owner of Houston's Texas Gallery, who was a regular at the original restaurant. "It wasn't Tex-Mex with yellow cheese and brown sauce. It was grilled meats with pico de gallo and fresh corn tortillas that they made on the premises. In 1973 these things were revolutionary." In retrospect, Ninfa's timing was perfect. The year before the first restaurant opened, Diana Kennedy had published her groundbreaking cookbook, *The Cuisines of Mexico*, and had caught the imagination of the entire country. Ninfa became a missionary for the more authentic style of Mexican cooking, and soon hundreds of customers were lining up on Friday nights for her incomparable *carnitas* and *tacos al carbón*.

But if Ninfa's was almost hysterically popular in the early years, it was not only because of Ninfa the savvy restaurateur. Much of that appeal came from Ninfa the woman. Her son Tom says, "Even when I was a teenager, my buddies would call her 'Mama.' People just automatically liked her." Her son-in-law Tony Mandola, the owner of Tony Mandola's Gulf Coast Kitchen, recalls that she was regarded as something of an oracle. "People would come in off the street and request a minute with Mama," he remembers, "not for business matters but for personal ones—marital difficulties, trouble with the children, health problems." Jackson Hicks, another longtime regular, felt that maternal aura: "She was a powerful woman, but it was a power that came from being centered on her family and clients. She made her customers—at least this customer—feel like they were family too."

Ninfa's restaurants hit hard times in the mid-nineties, with too-rapid expansion ending in a declaration of bankruptcy in 1996. Ninfa stayed on as a spokesperson for the chain after 1997, when it was bought by the Serranos restaurant group, but she could most often be found at her son Roland's restaurant, El Tiempo Cantina, laughing and smiling like in the old days. At her funeral, eulogists recalled her many community works, but Bishop Joseph Fiorenza summarized her legacy best when he spoke of her dedication to *la familia*. Mama Ninfa Laurenzo was everyone's mother.

*August 2001*

# JOHN MACKEY

EVAN SMITH

The 51-year-old co-founder and CEO of Whole Foods Market on profits, principles, chocolate-enrobed salmon, and why his wife won't play games with him anymore.

*On the way over to see you I passed the old Whole Foods location, at Tenth and Lamar [in Austin], and I got to thinking about how far you've come in the past couple of decades—not distancewise, since it's only a few blocks from there to the new, 80,000-square-foot store, but in terms of everything else.*

I'm less nostalgic about that location than the one that predated it—SaferWay, which was at Eighth and Rio Grande. It was the beginning of Whole Foods. My girlfriend and I started it. After two years we opened the store at Tenth and Lamar, and then we had a second store, and then a third and a fourth, but my memories of SaferWay are more intense. We literally lived in that store. We weren't supposed to, but we were buying stuff direct and putting it in the living room of the house we were renting; you'd come in the front door and you'd have to weave through all these bags of flour and rice and whatnot. Our landlord found out and gave us the boot. So then we said, "We're at the store all the time anyway. Why don't we just move into the third floor?" The story I love to tell is that we didn't have a shower. It was zoned commercial. So

*Evan*  we used to take baths in the Hobart dishwasher, which had a little
*Smith*  hose that hung down. And Barton Springs, of course.

*Could you ever have envisioned going from there to here? Was that
even your ambition?*

No, of course not. We started the business because, first, we
thought it would be fun. Second, we needed to earn a living, and
third, we wanted to earn a living in some way that we thought
would be beneficial to other people. We were young and idealistic.
I was 25, and she was 21—when you're young you don't know what
you can't do. If someone had said, "You're going to open a whole
bunch of stores and have a $4 billion company," I would have
thought that was the most ridiculous thing I had ever heard.

*Would it have upset or offended you? At a lot of companies founded
on principles, the notion of making money is almost antithetical to the
ethos of the place.*

From the very beginning our business has existed to meet the
needs and desires of multiple constituencies: customers, team
members, vendors, shareholders, the community. So I always
wanted to make money. I never thought profit was bad or evil. To
be sustainable, business has to be profitable. A business that is not
profitable is going to fail. At the same time, I've never felt comfortable with people who think the purpose of business is to make
a profit. That doesn't make any sense to me. It's like saying that
the purpose of life is to eat. Well, you can't live if you don't eat,
but you don't live to eat. And neither does business exist primarily to make a profit. It exists to fulfill its purpose, whatever that
might be.

*How did you learn how to do your job? Not everyone is born to run a
$4-billion company.*

There is no magic formula. I've learned, and I've grown by learning.
That's why I've enjoyed being in business so much: It's stretched
me. I've had to learn about myself, I've had to learn about other
people, and I've had to learn about how things work. I've always

seen it as a kind of game. I like games that are complex—the JOHN
deeper you get into the game, the more there is to learn. There's a MACKEY
stereotype out there in the world that businesspeople are stupid.
In fact, business is not simple. It's very difficult.

*What's the most difficult part?*

Every one of our stakeholders wants more. I can't go to a party
without somebody commenting on Whole Foods' prices—you
know, "Whole Paycheck," "You guys are so expensive"—and yet
our team members forever think they're underpaid. They're not
getting enough: "Look how rich and successful this company is."
Shareholders beat the drum for more profits and more growth.
The community's requests for donations are infinite. We give away
millions of dollars, but the more you give away, the more that people want you to give away. Then there's the government. Do you
know that when your company gets as large as Whole Foods, you
actually have to create office space for the IRS? They permanently
audit you.

My point is that the art of business is in some ways balancing so that everyone wins, so that everybody flourishes: customers
flourish, team members flourish, shareholders flourish, the community flourishes, government flourishes. But understand that
those balances are always temporary, because it's human nature
not to be satisfied for long. People want to know, "What have you
done for me lately?" You have to continue to rebalance as the business grows.

*Other than the "Whole Paycheck" example, are there other ways in
which you think the public's perception of the company doesn't square
with the way you see it?*

For ten, maybe fifteen years, I used to resent the fact that people
romanticize Whole Foods and unfairly project these aspirations
onto the company. I always wanted to shake them and say, "Gosh,
we're just a grocery store! We're not going to save the world!" And
then there are the people who just hate us. We've been attacked so
viciously. I've seen my name run into the dirt by the unions and
people on the left. I used to really resent it and resist it. And then

*Evan* I stopped resisting it. I got it. Whole Foods, for better or worse,
*Smith* is a very dynamic brand—it's very alive. And I don't think that's a
bad thing if we lead by example. With great power comes great responsibility. What the world wants business to do is to care about
more than just making money. And that's what business must
evolve to do.

*Why don't more companies understand that? Or is it that they do
understand but choose not to evolve?*

I'll tell you a story. When I speak at business schools, I start out
by saying, "How many people here think the purpose of business
is to maximize shareholder value?" Usually anywhere from a half
to two thirds of the room raise their hands. All of the professors
raise their hands. And then at the end of the speech, after I've
talked about creating a new paradigm, all of the students, or almost all of them, are super excited. They now have a vision of how
business could be noble. Business is usually the bad guy, but I've
given them a way to say, you know, business is the most transformative agency in the world, and they're the future leaders. They
can make money and do good. It's a very powerful message.

*Are the professors super excited too?*

They've got their arms crossed, because they think in terms of
black and white. They tend to think that you're either Mother
Teresa or Ken Lay. For some reason the idea of creating a win-
win scenario, that you can prosper and other people can prosper, doesn't come easy to them. That was the essential message of
Adam Smith in *The Wealth of Nations*. Our nation was founded
on similar principles: liberty leading to the collective good, the
notion that you can flourish but it doesn't have to come at the expense of anyone else—in fact, you can help them to flourish too.
The world needs to flourish. Humanity needs to flourish. So does
nature, the environment. And I think we can do it, but it's going to require business and business leadership to embrace a new
paradigm. The young people in these business schools are not yet
invested in the old paradigm, so when I say, "Hey, you can do well
and do good," the message resonates.

*Let's talk specifically about the grocery business. What got you
interested in it as opposed to something else?*

When I was growing up, my mother was totally fascinated by all
of the labor-saving devices like TV dinners and stuff you could get
in a can and open up and pour out and eat. For her it was a revolution, a release from the kind of cooking slavery that housewives
had endured for a long time. But to me, when I came of age, when
I became a young adult, it seemed like plastic food. It didn't seem
authentic. I was attracted to natural food because it was real. And
then I became aware that what you ate affected your health and
well-being and longevity and how you felt. And it was like, wow—
food raised the way it had been raised for thousands of years. Not
putting poisons on it. Not sticking a bunch of chemicals in it. Not
sticking it in cans.

The first natural-food store I ever walked into was a little co-
op in Austin. They had food in bulk bins. I'd never seen a whole
thing of rice before. Or barrels of beans. It was really exciting. I
joined the co-op and started to get interested in food, and then I
moved into a vegetarian co-op. The honest truth is that I wasn't a
vegetarian, but I thought, "I bet there are some really cool people
living in that co-op, and I bet there are some really cool women
living in that co-op." I was right on both counts. I learned how to
cook, and I got to be around people who were interested in the
same things I was beginning to get interested in, so I found peers.
I was alienated from society, and I wanted there to be a deeper
meaning to my life. Food is what I got into.

*You talk about "natural food," but some people think of Whole Foods
as a health-food store. Explain the difference.*

People don't like to create new categories. When we encounter
something genuinely new, we try to force it into an existing category, whether or not it fits. There was a health-food industry
that mostly sold vitamins and a kind of "superfood," food that
had magical powers. The idea was that if you took pills and ate
superfood, you'd be really healthy. The natural food movement,
which is where my roots are, thought, "No, not superfood—real
food, authentic food, whole food, food that's not technologically

altered." When science meets the organic, it begins to manipulate it, and not always in good ways. If you are trying to get into the real emotional, spiritual, psychological, philosophical energy that's behind the natural food movement, it's basically wanting food to be as natural and real and as minimally engineered and processed as possible.

*How involved are you these days in the minute details of the business?*

Not. Where I'm attached is the philosophy of the business. When I feel like someone is moving away from our mission, I dig my heels in and say no. If I feel like somebody is trying to undermine our culture, I say no.

*Give me an example.*

One of the co-founders of the company wanted us to sell cigarettes. And, in fact, one of our stores in Dallas sold them back in 1986.

*Did you know it at the time?*

No. Whole Foods has a policy that it's better to ask for forgiveness than permission. Part of our culture is to be forgiving. Try experiments. If it doesn't work, get rid of it.

*So selling cigarettes didn't work.*

Actually, it was working in terms of sales. They were selling American Spirits—natural tobacco. There are no artificial ingredients, no artificial flavorings, no added chemicals. The argument was, "Hey, we sell beer and wine. We sell ice cream. We sell things that aren't good for people. Why shouldn't we be able to sell this? We're not saying we should sell Marlboros, because they've got a bunch of chemicals in them. But these are natural cigarettes." There's a certain logic to that point of view. But, of course, the other point of view is that it completely contradicts the Whole Foods image. We had so many angry customers. They were mad because they had an image of Whole Foods in their minds. And now we weren't conforming to it anymore.

JOHN
MACKEY

*I wonder if the size of the new store will contradict that image as well.
I mean, who needs an 80,000-square-foot supermarket? Why is the
existing 35,000-square-foot store not good enough?*

When you see the new store, you'll know why. We're going to
have every kind of prepared food you can imagine. We're going to
have a much better salad bar than we have now. We'll have a pizza
oven. We'll have Chinese food, Indian food, Middle Eastern food,
Mexican food. We'll have a chocolate-enrobing station.

*A chocolate-enrobing station?*

This is a great example of how Whole Foods innovations occur.
You know how, on Valentine's Day, people dip strawberries in
chocolate? A local person at Whole Foods said, "Why don't we
do it all year?" So they started a little entrepreneurial chocolate-
dipping thing in one of our stores, and it was hugely successful.
Then we did it in our Columbus Circle store, in New York, and we
made a big deal out of it there.

*Just strawberries?*

No, anything. Even special orders.

*What if I want asparagus dipped in chocolate? No request too weird?*

No. Somebody asked for salmon to be enrobed, so they got
chocolate-enrobed salmon.

*How many of these decisions have been made based on what your
customers want versus what the competition is doing?*

Our most important stakeholder is the customer, so we're always
trying to figure out how to give the customer a better experience.

*Do you use focus groups?*

That's sort of top-down. The way our culture works is, we've got
166 stores, and every one of them is innovating and experiment-
ing. The team leader at every store can spend up to $100,000 a
year without asking for permission. We want them to try dif-

ferent things, and the things that are successful we'll study and copy and improve on. Most businesses have these command-and-control models. McDonald's is the best example of that. They're cookie cutters. They have a formula that works. Don't surprise the customers. Give them exactly what they expect. Make it consistent. It's the mass-market football model of executing the game plan—don't fumble the ball, don't make any mistakes. Whole Foods is more like a fast-breaking basketball team. We're driving down the court, but we don't exactly know how the play is going to evolve.

*So you don't care at all about the competition? You don't care that the flagship Central Market, in Austin, just massively retooled in a way that seems to have your new store in its sights?*

I never said I don't care about the competition. I'm a very competitive person. There are times when my wife won't play games with me, for example. A lot of people don't want to be my partner in card games because I'm very intense and I want to win. But I like it when competitors do things that are innovative. If we get an idea from them, we can spread it around to our whole company. If we steal something from Central Market in Austin and it shows up in our Chicago stores, we're better off as a result, and so are our customers.

*Do you ever shop at Central Market?*

Of course not.

*Why not?*

It's a matter of principle. Can you see how it would play in the newspapers?

*Wait a minute. What if you were an executive at an airline that doesn't fly everywhere? Are you not going to travel to those places? Or are you going to suck it up and hop on another airline?*

There is nothing I eat that I can't get at Whole Foods.

*Have you ever had a disappointing experience shopping at one of your own stores?*

Of course.

*Tell me a specific story.*

Maybe the cashier is talking to the bagger instead of paying attention to the customer. That is completely against the philosophy of the business.

*Do you ever say anything?*

Not directly to them, which would be inappropriate. What I would do instead is talk to the shift manager or the store team leader—not to be a tattletale but to indicate that this was going on in their store, so that they would pay more attention to it. I've been doing this for 27 years. I can go into a store and tell you within five minutes if that store is well managed or not, if the morale is good or not, if the store is clean or not. They may have known I was coming, but it won't make any difference. I can feel it; I can see it. But I'm very aware that what the team members mostly want from me is my approval. I am a father figure. I'm a daddy. There's no other way to put it. So when I go into our stores, I really try to focus on what we're doing right. It's not my job to focus on what we're doing wrong.

*March 2005*

# JOHN CAMPBELL

## PATRICIA SHARPE

<big>H</big>is appetite for marketing revolutionized the way we shop for groceries.

I WAS LOITERING AROUND the newest Central Market in Austin on a Sunday afternoon not long ago, killing time while the in-house cafe prepared my roasted-vegetable Slacker Sandwich, when I noticed them: The People Without Shopping Carts. They were a group of four, a young couple in their twenties and a set of middle-aged parents. First they inspected the awesome *affinage*, a climate-controlled vault where you can buy and age your own, personal piece of Spenwood sheep's-milk cheese or Montgomery's cheddar. Next they wandered over to the open bakery, where a fresh, hot loaf of pistachio-fig bread had been cut up for sampling. Then they headed to the produce department to ooh and aah over the twenty varieties of apples and the trendy Dolce Mediterraneo peppers. When I stopped tailing them, the foursome was in the toiletries section, sniffing the $6.79 bars of French-milled soap. They never bought a thing and never intended to. They were sightseers on the Austin tourist trail, which in the past five years has come to include—along with the state capitol, Barton Springs, and the LBJ Library—Central Market.

In January 1994 this division of San Antonio–based H-E-B broke new ground in grocery retailing. It threw out the one-stop-shopping model—getting rid of all the boring, oppressive shelves of dog food, toilet paper, and breakfast cereal—and launched a breezy, accessible, subtly upscale store that focused exclusively on food, food, food. In the five years and nine months since then, Central Market has become famous in the supermarket industry as well as among people who live to eat. Stories have appeared in the *Wall Street Journal, Self,* and *Better Homes and Gardens,* among other publications. Kate Krader, a *Food & Wine* magazine senior editor, calls the market "phenomenal." Ron Lieber, who wrote about it for the slick business magazine *Fast Company,* says, "It's the coolest grocery store I've ever seen."

Since the initial store opened, two more Central Markets have followed—one in San Antonio in 1998 and the second Austin store in April of this year. The concept has such cachet that H-E-B is looking to expand it (a site is being sought in Houston; Dallas will probably come next). But if you asked the hordes of shoppers pawing through the portobellos and porcinis to name the individual who turned the idea into reality, not one in a hundred would be able to tell you that the credit belongs to a modest, affable 48-year-old corporate vice president named John Campbell.

Campbell is an unlikely person to have made grocery shopping sexy. Indeed, in his conservative polo shirt and khaki pants, he looks every inch the company man and accountant that he is. He started out as a sacker at a Corpus Christi H-E-B when he was a kid and climbed the corporate ladder into upper-level administration. In thirty years, incredibly, he never left the fold. But if Campbell doesn't fit the model of the freewheeling entrepreneur, he has attributes that are even more valuable for trail-bossing a new operation: deep experience and natural leadership. In late 1992—a year after the Central Market idea began to percolate in the minds of H-E-B chairman and CEO Charles Butt, president Fully Clingman, and a core group of other executives—Campbell was tapped to head the development team. "They thought I was crazy enough to take it on," he says. Butt saw other qualities: "John has a roster of food friendships all over the country, and he is out there on the cutting edge about products. He also attracted a group of truly talented people to work for him. Of all the reasons for his success, I'd say that is number one, two, and three."

Campbell made Central Market his baby. To check out the

best ideas in food retailing, a task force of senior managers began making extensive visits to stores all over North America and Europe. Harry's Farmers Market in Atlanta showed them how to capture the nostalgic appeal of an old-time fruit-and-vegetable stand in a modern produce emporium. Mexico City's flower and food markets dazzled them with their bounty and beauty. In an open-air market in Belgium, Campbell remembers, "We saw a hundred different kinds of dressed olives—I mean, it was breathtaking." On one 2-week trip to Europe, the group visited 74 stores in thirteen cities in seven countries. Closer to home, they looked at Austin-based Whole Foods Market's way with bins of grains and spices. "Not knowing what would work and what would flop—that was scary," he says. But in the end, it all came together. The Austin Central Market had revenues of between $40 million and $50 million in 1998, with a profit margin of around 1 percent—quite respectable in the grocery business. Campbell, who had only intended to open a new store, had created a new model for grocery retailing.

While one might naturally expect the Central Market concept to be rapidly cloned across H-E-B's U.S. territory of Texas and Louisiana, Campbell says, "These stores are so talent-intensive that you can't do one on demand. It has to be customized for each location, and it takes a powerful team to make one work." He recently hired two graduates of Cornell University's business management school and is getting them ready to come online. But even though it won't be easy to open the new stores, the experience won't be nearly as stomach churning as that first dive off the high board five years ago. As Campbell says, "Nobody ever asked for a Central Market." He took something that we didn't know we needed and he made it indispensable.

*September 1999*

# GOT GAME

PATRICIA SHARPE

Hudson's on the Bend is where Austinites (and foodies from near and far) go wild for smoked venison and other full-flavored fare. With these recipes, you can too.

SEVERAL YEARS AGO MY MOTHER phoned me with an urgent question. "Honey, I need your advice on something," she said. Resisting the impulse to shout, "Omigod, hell has frozen over!" I replied, "Sure, what is it?" Her query, as it turned out, was easy: Where should she and Daddy take the family to celebrate their forty-ninth wedding anniversary?

Without hesitating, I said, "Hudson's on the Bend." The rustic domain of chef-owner Jeff Blank has been one of my favorite Austin restaurants since it opened twenty years ago near Hudson Bend, a small community on a curve of Lake Travis. In my opinion, it is *the* default local choice for anniversaries, proposals, and schmoozing the boss.

The menu is appropriately Texas-centric, with influences from the diverse ethnic groups that settled this part of the state as well as cowboys and hunters. And the fact that the charming converted house is a thirty-minute drive from town makes it seem as if you're going somewhere special. Fresh herbs grow in the garden you pass on your way in, tiny lights twinkle in the live oaks you glimpse from the low-slung, limestone-walled rooms, and if you're dining on the patio, you might catch a whiff of smoke from the grill, upon which is certain to be a haunch of wild game or a sumptuous array of seafood, the dual specialties of the kitchen.

To celebrate having survived two decades in the restaurant business—a feat akin to winning the Tour de France six times—this month Hudson's is publishing its second cookbook, *Fired Up! More Adventures and Recipes From Hudson's on the Bend* (Laurentius Press, 2005), with a foreword by loyal customer Lance Armstrong. In it you'll find the secrets for preparing iconic dishes like the ones here: Hill Country peach-and-goat-cheese salad, smoked venison in Shiner Bock "beer blanc," and grilled summer squash with "avomole." Assisted by a round of Blank's basil mojitos, they'll satisfy your soul on a sultry Texas day.

## BASIL MOJITO

> 1 lime, halved lengthwise
> 2 ounces (¼ cup) simple syrup (consult a cookbook for
>     instructions) or 3 teaspoons sugar
> 10 fresh basil leaves plus a sprig for garnish
> ½ cup ice
> 1 to 1 ½ounces rum
> 2 ounces (¼ cup) club soda

Squeeze half the lime into a tall glass. Cut other half into 4 wedges and put 3 in the glass. Add simple syrup and basil leaves and muddle to extract flavor. Add ice, rum, and club soda; stir. Garnish with basil sprig and remaining lime wedge. Makes 1 drink.

## HILL COUNTRY PEACH SALAD WITH
## SPICY CANDIED PECANS

### Balsamic-Apple Vinaigrette

> 2 cups balsamic vinegar
> ½ tablespoon apple juice concentrate (available in frozen
>     foods section)

In a nonreactive saucepan over high heat, reduce vinegar to a syrup-like consistency (about ¾ cup), lowering heat to a simmer when volume is around 1 cup; test consistency by removing a spoonful and letting it cool (process takes about 35 minutes). Cool to room temperature and stir in concentrate. Transfer to a squirt bottle.

### Salad

2 egg whites
1 tablespoon Grand Marnier
½ teaspoon salt
1 ½ cups powdered sugar
1 to 2 tablespoons cayenne pepper
4 cups pecan halves
8 ripe peaches
12 ounces goat cheese (Hudson's uses Pure Luck brand chèvre)

Make candied pecans: Preheat oven to 350 degrees. In a mixing bowl, beat or whisk egg whites until foamy. Add Grand Marnier and whisk again. Mix salt, sugar, and cayenne pepper together and whisk into egg-white mixture, blending thoroughly. Gently fold pecans into mixture until coated. Spread on a cookie sheet lined with parchment paper and bake for 15 minutes. Remove from oven and stir to break up. Return to oven for 15 more minutes. Let cool before using. When ready to make salad, pit peaches (peel if you wish) and slice into wedges ½- to ¾-inch thick. Arrange wedges in pinwheels on 8 plates and sprinkle candied pecans and dollops of goat cheese around them. Then find your inner Jackson Pollock and drizzle salad with Balsamic-Apple Vinaigrette. Serves 8.

## ESPRESSO-RUBBED VENISON WITH SHINER BOCK "BEER BLANC"

### Beer Blanc

12 ounces Shiner Bock or any bock beer
2 shallots, finely chopped
2 cloves garlic, finely chopped
2 canned chipotle chiles, seeded if you wish and chopped
¼ cup heavy cream
juice of 1 lime
2 sticks butter, cut into 1-inch pieces, at room temperature
salt and white pepper

*Patricia*
*Sharpe* In a saucepan over medium heat, reduce beer to ¼ cup (takes 35 to 40 minutes). Add shallots, garlic, chipotles, and cream and simmer until volume is reduced by half. Add lime juice and continue heating until liquid returns to a simmer. While mixture is still very hot, pour into a blender and purée, adding butter one piece at a time. Season to taste. If not using immediately, keep hot in an insulated container such as a thermal pitcher.

## Venison

¼ cup finely ground espresso coffee beans
1 tablespoon sea salt
½ teaspoon ancho chile powder
½ teaspoon freshly ground black pepper
2 pounds venison backstrap or pork tenderloin
lump crabmeat, cooked (optional)

Note: Venison is available from Whole Foods and Central Market (may require advance order) or by mail from Broken Arrow Ranch, in Ingram (830-367-5871; brokenarrowranch.com). You will need a stove-top smoker such as the approximately 15-inch-by-11-inch one made by Camerons, available from Central Market, cookingfearlessly.com/store.htm (the Hudson's website), or amazon.com. It comes with wood chips, but feel free to use different woods such as apple or pear or throw in a sprig of fresh rosemary or other herb you would enjoy. Smokers may be used on gas or electric ranges; if you have a flattop electric stove, consult smoker's instruction manual.

Thoroughly combine first 4 ingredients. Coat meat with mixture an hour before smoking. Pile about 2 tablespoons of wood chips in middle of smoker pan. Place smoker drip tray over chips and put the wire rack on top of it. (Hint: To aid cleanup, spray rack with vegetable oil and spray tray as well or cover it with foil.) Put venison on rack.

Slide lid closed and center smoker on a stove burner over high heat. The wood chips will slowly burn, smoking the venison as it cooks. Continue cooking until an instant-read meat thermometer inserted in middle of venison reads 130 degrees, 15 to 18 minutes

(140 degrees, 18 to 20 minutes for pork). Remove meat and let rest for 5 to 10 minutes, then cut into ½-inch slices. Fan 3 slices across each plate and top with Beer Blanc and crabmeat. Serves 6 to 8.

## GRILLED SUMMER SQUASH WITH "AVOMOLE"

### Avomole Sauce

5 tomatillos, husks removed
2 jalapeños, seeded if you wish
3 ripe avocados
1 cup roughly chopped white onion
½ bunch cilantro, large stems cut off
½ cup heavy cream
juice of 2 limes
salt to taste

Blanch tomatillos and jalapeños in boiling water for 2 minutes, then immediately plunge into ice water to retain bright green color. Put all ingredients in a blender and purée.

### Squash

6 summer squash (yellow crookneck, pattypan, zucchini) or
    chayotes or a mixture
½ cup extra-virgin olive oil
salt and freshly ground black pepper
3 or 4 limes

Heat grill to medium. Cut squash into 1-inch slices and place on skewers. Brush with olive oil and season liberally. Grill for 3 or 4 minutes, turning several times, until tender but not overdone.

To serve, put several spoonfuls of Avomole on each plate. (You will have sauce left over.) Squeeze limes on squash and place a skewer of squash on top of sauce. Serves 6 to 8.

*July 2005*

# STEPHAN PYLES

### PATRICIA SHARPE

The star of Southwestern cuisine is taking his toque on the road.

IN THE RAREFIED WORLD OF SUPERCHEFS, Stephan Pyles is a player. The trim, neatly bearded fifth-generation Texan is the creator of two of Dallas's most lionized restaurants—frontier-sleek Star Canyon and splashy, Caribbean-cool Aqua-Knox. He has written or coauthored four cookbooks and is the star of his own cooking series on public television. He helped invent Southwestern cuisine and is in demand for lavish charity dinners and cooking classes all over; the big wall-calendar outside his office has notes like "S.P. in Spain" and "S.P. in Mexico." When he has a few spare days to just hang out, he can call up hotshot chef pals like Mark Miller of Santa Fe's Coyote Cafe and John Sedlar of Abiquiu in San Francisco. Not bad for a kid who started out rolling tamales at his parents' Big Spring truck stop.

But being a player is one thing; being a Player with a capital *P* is another, and six months ago the 45-year-old chef's already high profile took a decidedly uppercase turn. In March, Carlson Companies—a $20 billion Minneapolis-based group whose subsidiaries own nearly a hundred corporations around the world, including Radisson Hotels and T.G.I. Friday's—bought Star Canyon and AquaKnox from Pyles and his two partners. The selling price was a secret, though the two sophisticated restaurants are expected to gross $10 million this year. The plan is to take them international, with Carlson providing the wherewithal. Pyles will stay in place as chef at large and mother hen of the expansion and will also generate new concepts, such as a string of Mexican *taquerías* already on the drawing board. For his part, Pyles seems exhilarated at the new opportunity if a bit exhausted by the negotiations: His face, wreathed in smiles, twitches ever so slightly as we talk. Right now he's fretting because some customers and a local food columnist have voiced fears that he'll never pick up a whisk again. "I understand that people take Star Canyon to heart and think of it as their own place, and they're afraid it has gone commercial," he says. "We'll have to prove to them that we can expand and still keep the quality up." If all goes according to plan, in five years travelers to Las Vegas, Chicago, Orlando, London, and Hong Kong could well be dining at Star Canyons or AquaKnoxes (although the latter's name, with its reference to Dallas's Knox Street, may be changed for other cities). Ventures in Sydney and Paris are not out of the question.

In the midst of all the hoopla and hype, no one seems to have noticed the quiet revolution that has occurred: Thanks in large part to Pyles, the term "Texas cuisine" is no longer an oxymoron. Though Texas food has never lacked for brand-name recognition, the restaurants that have served it nationally have tended to be of the yeehaw variety: Lone Star Cafe, Texas Land and Cattle Company, Chili's. High-level, innovative Texas cooking has been concentrated primarily at restaurants in Dallas and Houston and thus has been mainly for local consumption. Carlson Companies' move changes that equation. "Texas will always have that Western cachet; there's just an aura about it," says Pyles. "But Texas is a far more sophisticated place than it was twenty years ago."

In the year 2000, when customers in Chicago open one of Star Canyon's big leather-bound menus, their horizons and their notion of Texas cuisine will expand. They will of course find the restaurant's fantastic, mammoth Cowboy Ribeye, but there will also be Pyles' silky salmon in a hot-sweet chile-molasses glaze with a plantain–sweet potato mash on the side and his rosy seared duck breast with a savory herbed bread pudding jazzed up by pumpkin seeds. Patrons at the London edition of AquaKnox will discover the likes of lemongrass prawns with a purple sticky rice tamale

and coconut curry sauce. Texas cooking of a certain level has en-
tered the global arena, something that was not imaginable a generation ago, and Stephan Pyles has done a lot to make it happen.
These days when people talk about Texas food, the conversation
may begin at the barbecue pit, but it definitely does not end there.

*September 1998*